BY TASNEEM BHATIA, M.D.

The 21-Day Belly Fix

What Doctors Eat

The 21-Day Belly Fix

THE 21-DAY
BELLY
FIX

The Doctor-Designed
Diet Plan for a Clean Gut
and a Slimmer Waist

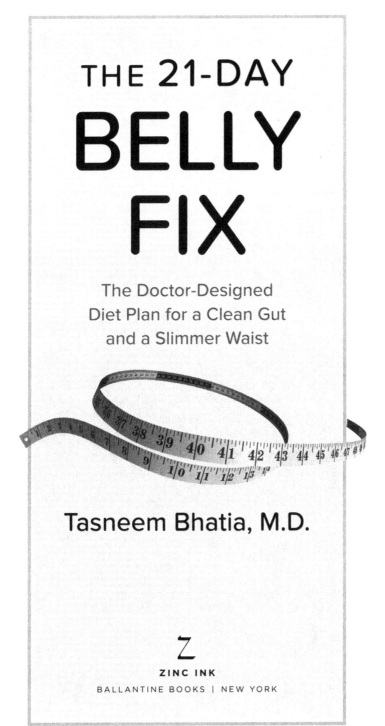

Tasneem Bhatia, M.D.

Z

ZINC INK

BALLANTINE BOOKS | NEW YORK

This book proposes a program of diet and exercise recommendations for the reader to follow. However, you should consult a qualified medical professional (including, if you are pregnant, your ob-gyn) before starting this or any other fitness program. Please seek your doctor's advice before making any decisions that affect your health or extreme changes in your diet, particularly if you suffer from any medical condition or have any symptom that may require treatment. As with any diet or exercise program, if at any time you experience any discomfort, stop immediately and consult your physician.

A Zinc Ink Trade Paperback Original

Copyright © 2014 by Dr. Tasneem Bhatia

Published in the United States by Zinc Ink,
an imprint of Random House, a division of Random House LLC,
a Penguin Random House Company, New York.

BALLANTINE and the HOUSE colophon are
registered trademarks of Random House LLC.

ZINC INK is a trademark of David Zinczenko.

LIBRARY OF CONGRESS CATALOGING-IN-PUBLICATION DATA
Bhatia, Tasneem.
The 21-day belly fix: the doctor-designed diet plan
for a clean gut and a slimmer waist / Tasneem Bhatia, M.D.
pages   cm
title: Twenty-one-day belly fix
Includes bibliographical references and index.
ISBN 978-0-553-39364-4
eBook ISBN 978-0-553-39363-7
1. Weight loss. 2. Reducing diets. 3. Reducing exercises. 4. Digestive organs—
Diseases—Treatment. I. Title. II. Title: Twenty-one-day belly fix.
RM222.2.B52 2014
613.2'5—dc23   2014029114

Printed in the United States of America on acid-free paper

www.ballantinebooks.com

2 4 6 8 9 7 5 3 1

Book design by Casey Hampton

Writing this book was an act of pure joy because I was finally able to share my years of research and experience with you, the reader. I could not have done it without the help of both Julia Vantine and Rachel Meltzer Warren, M.S., R.D.N., who forced me daily to get my thoughts together. I want to thank my family for putting up with my crazy work and writing schedules, especially my sweet husband, Vik, and our children, Rania and Kubby. Finally, this book could not have been written without my patients, who ultimately are my teachers and force me to be better every day.

Tasneem Bhatia, M.D.

Contents

Introduction

"It shouldn't be this hard for me to lose weight."

I hear this time and again from first-time patients. Often they have seen doctor after doctor before they arrive at my practice, which is one of the country's leading holistic and integrative medical centers. More often than not, they don't know why they can't drop the pounds, despite their strenuous diet and exercise regimens. Equally confused are those who come to me with allergies, rashes, depression, migraines, overwhelming fatigue, or inability to conceive: Their specialists don't have any answers, either.

I'll never forget the day that one particularly frustrated patient walked into my office for the first time. My clinic, on a tree-lined street in Atlanta, is a warm place, with soft lighting, light music, and aromatherapy—earth tones dominate, so patients feel comfortable. It's a safe space, and I encourage a dialogue. It's not unusual for people to bring in their medical records, lists of medications, x-rays, and bags of supplements they're taking. This patient, however, was unique. She brought in a stack of books—diet books.

"I have tried them all," she declared in frustration, "and none have worked. I have fasted, detoxed, 'gone Paleo'—nothing is working. I'm now fifty pounds overweight, and I have gained it all in the last three years!"

Concerned, I looked at her critically. She was in her late forties, her face was puffy and swollen, she had dark circles under her eyes, and most of her weight was centered in her abdomen. I understood her frustration—day after day, patient after patient, I am asked about weight and how to lose it. And I have the vantage point of seeing everyone—the active mom who wants to lose that last five pounds, the busy executive who has had too many business dinners, and the severely overweight, whose lifelong struggles have led to chronic diseases like diabetes, hypertension, metabolic syndrome, and cancer.

The struggle to shed weight has become an American story, with all of us affected, either personally or through a loved one fighting that battle.

I always listen quietly. But as I review their health questionnaires, ask follow-up questions about their diet and lifestyle, and perform their physical exams, I say the same thing time and again: "Let's start with your gut."

Here's what I know: Nine times out of ten, my patients are "in the gutter"—my term for experiencing the effects of an out-of-whack digestive system.

Weight gain begins in the gut, and we now have the research to prove it. Altered gut microbiology—the wrong bacteria, yeast, or a damaged gut lining—leads to extra pounds. How? Well, for one, sugar cravings, carbohydrate addiction, and the desire for high-fat foods all begin in the belly: When our gut is damaged, our neurotransmitters are affected, making our body respond in kind. Carbs help give us a quick burst of serotonin, fats help us manage dopamine and norepinephrine, and sugar quickly boosts insulin and cortisol. And that's why you reach for the Krispy Kremes. These quick fixes work, for a moment—until your body craves more, and you start the cycle all over again.

Let's go back to my patient with all her books. She had dieted, experimenting with different plans, and also alternated between starving and bingeing. The psychological toll of gaining weight triggered a depression, and she started isolating herself. Her clothes did not fit, and she was too ashamed to buy new ones.

Like many other patients, she had been approaching weight loss the wrong way. Diet and exercise do indeed help, but only if your gut, your hormones, and your stress levels are managed appropriately.

Together, we decided on starting the 21-Day Belly Fix, to begin rehabbing her belly as an initial step for weight loss. Following our plan, she removed gluten, lowered her sugar intake, and provided her belly with digestive enzymes, probiotics, and berberine—an herb I often use to treat candida, a fungus in the belly.

After her twenty-one days, she lost ten pounds, improved her insulin regulation, and noticed that her energy had increased dramatically. By sixty days, she had lost twenty-one pounds. A year later I saw her in the office, and she is back to her original size 6.

She got there not by dieting but by *fixing* her diet. She got there thanks to the 21-Day Belly Fix. And now, with this book, you can get there, too.

DIET-FREE WEIGHT LOSS? REALLY?

Yes, it's possible, with the 21-Day Belly Fix. The secret is in changing your gut's bacteria, making sure there's more "good" than "bad." By doing so, you'll not only lose weight and feel better, but you'll also be at the forefront of a new movement. You may have seen the recent headlines: "Bacteria in the Intestines May Help Tip the Bathroom Scale, Studies Show," touted the *New York Times* last year. "The Humble Heroes of Weight-Loss Surgery: Stomach Acids and Gut Microbes," trumpeted *National Geographic* this past March. "Increasingly, scientists, physicians, and the public are recognizing that the gut microbiota, the microbes that live within our intestines, shape our health and wellbeing in innumerable ways," reported the Harvard School of Public Health last year.

Gut health is hot right now. And for good reason: Gut health is *the key* to good health—and to losing weight.

On the 21-Day Belly Fix, you'll lose 10 pounds at least during the plan alone. But I call it "diet-free weight loss," because you'll continue to feel great long afterward due to your newly balanced bacteria. As a result, you will:

LOSE WEIGHT Your bacteria—not your lack of willpower!—may be responsible for your weight gain. Just last year, researchers found that a natural enzyme that keeps bad gut bacteria in check may be able to prevent obesity—and may be able to reverse it. Another study, from researchers at Cedars-Sinai Medical Center in Los Angeles, found that people with a greater amount of methane gas in their bodies—from methane gas bacteria—digested their food more slowly and thus were gaining more weight than other people without even knowing it. Yes, *without even knowing it!* The whole premise of the 21-Day Belly Fix is to rebalance your gut bacteria so that your gut can help you burn calories, not add more!

REDUCE INFLAMMATION When the Harvard School of Public Health wrote that "the microbes that live within our intestines shape our health and wellbeing in innumerable ways," they were referring specifically to a report that found that "chemicals generated by bacteria in the colon help important immune cells," which reduced inflammation in mice. That means your irritable bowel syndrome, your bloating, your excess gas—it could all be caused by the *wrong bacteria* in your gut.

SPEED UP METABOLISM This was big news last year: Scientists took two twin mice—one obese, one thin—and transplanted their gut bacteria into sterile mice. "The lean bugs went into the obese community, transforming it," said Jeffrey Gordon, a microbiologist and director of the Center of Genome Science and Systems Biology at the Washington University School of Medicine in St. Louis. Meanwhile, the thin ones "increased the amount of fat in their body." The findings established a direct link between your bacteria and how quickly you burn fat.

HELP YOUR DEPRESSION You usually think of depression starting in your head. But if you're feeling low (and eating more as a result), the reason may be your gut. New research proves that altering your gut's bacteria could influence your behavior: Mice with good belly bacteria were found to be less anxious in a recent study in *Proceedings of the National Academy of Sciences,* and I've seen the link in my own patients time and again. There's a "brain" in your gut, and in *The 21-Day Belly Fix,* I'll show you how to control it.

These findings are the result of years of research by scientists. But I've witnessed the healing effects firsthand for more than decade, and I'm ready to share my secret with you. As you can see, the 21-Day Belly Fix won't just help you stay thin. If you're plagued by mystery symptoms that impact your quality of life—depression, hair loss, diabetes—you, like my patients, are likely in the gutter. Many, many people end up there—even physicians. Even me.

"YOU NEED TO CLEAN YOUR BELLY"

I was twenty-eight, working as an ER physician in Atlanta, and sick—with what, I didn't know. The onset of my symptoms was gradual but had grown steadily worse. No obvious digestive-system problems, but my hair was falling out, my skin was erupting with cystic acne, and my periods were irregular. I exercised aggressively but could not lose weight and was ten pounds heavier than I am today.

I didn't yet know about the gut/health connection, and neither did the specialists I consulted. Each followed the same script. Step one: Run tests. Allergy tests. Blood tests. A biopsy of my scalp, which was quite painful.

None could offer a diagnosis. My symptoms were not "severe" enough, they said. Seriously? I was having my period once every two or three months. My hair was clogging the drain after every shower. That wasn't "severe"?

The lack of a diagnosis didn't stop them from proceeding to Step Two: Prescribe meds. The gynecologist wanted me on birth control pills to regulate my cycle. The dermatologist wanted me on a medication prescribed to men with enlarged prostates—and prescribed off-label to women with hair loss. This is a medication so potent that women who are pregnant or of childbearing age aren't even supposed to touch it.

Remember, I was twenty-eight. "If you don't take it, young lady, you'll be bald within a few years," the well-known, world-renowned dermatologist warned.

My allergist had nothing. My test results showed no allergies to either environmental allergens (things like dust and ragweed) or common foods like wheat or dairy. "Your diet has nothing to do with your symptoms," she said. I thanked her and left.

Unsatisfied and irritated didn't begin to describe my feeling about the treatment options I'd been offered. I felt lost. What was causing my symptoms? What was my body trying to tell me? Finding the answers would take almost a decade—and change the course of my health, my career, and my life purpose. The book you're holding, *The 21-Day Belly Fix,* is the result of that epic journey.

After three years of frustration and increasing alienation from my mainstream medical training, I began to study nutrition, alternative medicine systems, and holistic medicine, which treat the whole person in body, mind, and spirit.

In 2003, I was board-certified in holistic medicine and became a certified nutrition specialist in 2004. My studies had expanded my understanding of health and disease far beyond what I'd learned in medical school. But there *was* still more to learn. In 2006, I left Atlanta and headed to San Francisco to study Chinese medicine. Six years had passed since the onset of my symptoms, and my health puzzle was not yet solved. It was time to dig deeper.

My conventional training had taught me to meet symptoms with force—suppression is the goal. Now Chinese medicine was teaching me a different tack: healing the root causes of disease in addition to treating symptoms. Prevent symptoms, rather than react to them. How refreshing! The approach felt right to me.

One day, as we practiced diagnosing each other Chinese-medicine-style, the head professor—a small Asian man in his mid-seventies, bespectacled and stooped—stopped at my table, regarding me intently. Taking a seat across from mine, he peered into my face, looked carefully at my tongue, and took my pulse. His whole body seemed to be listening to mine. I could feel his mind probing for weakness, for imbalance. Nervous, I held my breath.

Finally, he sat back. "Young lady," he said, in heavily accented English. "You have a very bad gut. Too much, too much dampness. You need to clean your belly."

My *gut*? What was he talking about? None of my previous medical training had connected tortured skin, thinning hair, and missing-in-action periods to an unhealthy digestive system. But something told me that he was right.

My diet had to change, he said. I couldn't argue. For years now—all through the grind of medical school, residency, and twelve- and fourteen-hour shifts at the ER—"eating" meant peeling a wrapper or opening a box or bag. Processed food. Fast food. Junk. I would learn that sugar, grease, and white flour are the building blocks of a "damp diet." Even the *way* I was eating had promoted dampness. I either skipped meals or choked them down on the run.

My teacher prescribed a regimen of dietary changes and herbs to give my overburdened belly a rest. While it didn't magically resolve my symptoms, I began to feel better, to sleep better, to lose weight. I felt confident that I was on the right track. As my diet improved, I learned more about the power of nutrition and how it related to my symptoms. That study led me right back to the digestive system. I used my training in nutrition and traditional and Western systems of medicine to diagnose hypothyroidism and gluten sensitivity, a condition that occurs when you ingest a protein found in wheat, rye, barley, and a few other grains. Gluten intolerance can cause belly symptoms, like bloating and abdominal pain, as well as joint pain and depression. Again, these conditions circled back to the gut.

PHYSICIAN, HEALING HERSELF

During this healing period, my hair loss stopped, my skin cleared up, and my periods began to arrive each month and on time. I also married, completed a fellowship in integrative medicine at the University of Arizona in Tucson, had my children, and founded the Atlanta Center for Holistic and Integrative Medicine. By this time, fully healed, I was using the knowledge I'd gained from my own recovery to heal my patients. I still do.

I love what I do, and my practice just keeps growing. But why? I think its success suggests a frustration with mainstream medicine, which focuses on managing symptoms rather than getting to their roots. That's what medical school and residency trained me to do. That's what the specialists who initially treated me did. Mainstream physicians are taught to be reactive: For Symptom X, take or do Y.

But the human body isn't a flow chart. It's a dynamic organism. Its systems—cardiovascular, endocrine, reproductive, lymphatic, respiratory— are designed to work in harmony.

Above all, the body seeks balance. (*Homeostasis,* to use the medical term.) A disturbance in one system ripples through others. Ailments of the body affect the mind and emotions. And ailments of the mind, including stress, anxiety, and depression, promote disease, in large part by disrupting our self-care. We eat and sleep too much or too little, stop moving our bodies, chain-smoke, abuse alcohol, all of which undermines our physical health. Some of us take the opposite approach—read every health book, search Doctor Google to self-diagnose every health issue, jump into the latest fad diet.

Many mainstream physicians pay lip service to the mind-body connection, but not many walk the walk. They tell their patients to lose weight but not how to nourish their bodies. They advise stress management but aren't familiar with ancient relaxation techniques vetted by science. I believe that America's dismal state of health care (including exorbitant expenditures) stem from mainstream medicine's dismissal of traditional healing systems that counter the Western definitions of health and disease. These systems, thousands of years old, use vastly different (and decidedly low-tech) diagnostic tools. Even stranger to the Western model: They focus on vitality rather than disease.

Mainstream medicine's dismissal of alternative medicine systems

5 Reasons You're in the Gutter

Powered by junk food and stress, the Western lifestyle is putting the whammy on the American gut. Here are some of the top belly offenders.

Our nutrient-poor diet. Laden with sugar, fat, and refined grains, our junk-food diet discourages the microbial diversity that the digestive system requires for health. A century ago, people ate seasonally—what was growing in the ground in spring, summer, or fall ended up on their plates. Modern farming practices use less crop rotation and more chemicals, which deplete the soil of essential nutrients and microbes. Also, eating the same foods over and over (even healthy ones) or eating mostly processed foods creates an altered gut microbiology that can trigger inflammation and promote a leaky gut.

Mass-produced food. Yogurt in a tube. Frozen dinners. Ravioli in a can. Rotgut, all of it. Big Food has contributed to the disappearance of microbial diversity, triggering leaky guts and inflammation. Consider a common staple: packaged sandwich bread. Our grandmothers and great grandmothers made homemade bread from dough that was allowed to rise for a good long time. The longer bread dough ferments, the more varied bacteria it will contain.

Packaged bread has no microbial diversity. It may also be made with hybridized wheat—the price one pays for wheat that grows faster and resists drought and insects. Hybridized wheat contains new proteins not found in the earliest wheat strains. These new proteins may be playing a part in the rise of gluten intolerance and celiac disease.

Overuse of certain medications. Over-the-counter or prescription acid blockers, non-steroidal anti-inflammatory drugs (NSAIDs) such as common pain relievers, and overuse of antibiotics can damage the gut's intestinal lining.

Undiagnosed food allergies. Allergies to foods such as dairy, eggs, or corn can affect the gut, as can an intolerance to gluten.

Stress. Unmanaged chronic stress can contribute to an imbalance of gut bacteria and contribute to a leaky gut. And it can also cause changes in the gut's nervous system.

borders on arrogance. And yet, among my colleagues, there's a quiet acknowledgment that million-dollar medical technologies and hundred-dollar pills have had a less-than-stellar success rate.

For me, the beauty of integrative medicine is that *this* system of medicine combines the best of *all* systems of medicine. I can take from them all and make an accurate diagnosis. And 75 percent of the time, it's gut-related.

GET THE GUTS TO BE HEALTHY

Once upon a time, everyone knew that the gut is the gateway to health. Hippocrates, the father of modern medicine, knew it, uttering that famous aphorism, "All disease begins in the gut." American physician, health-food pioneer, and breakfast-cereal scion John Harvey Kellogg preached the healing power of good digestion, a vegetarian diet, and regular exercise. (Immortalized in the novel and film *The Road to Wellville,* Kellogg was also something of a kook, with some ideas that, it must be said, went too far.)

But over time, we've largely forgotten the gut's connection to health. As mainstream medicine became more and more fragmented and doctors started to specialize in just one system of the body, we lost sight of the holistic big picture. Our Western lifestyle compounds this oversight. A steady diet of processed food, chronic stress, medication overuse, chemicals in the air and water . . . all of these place a toxic burden on the gut. While we love our modern conveniences, the remote and the drive-through ushered in a new set of illnesses and an overweight but malnourished population.

And here we are. Fighting extra pounds and fatigue. Popping pain relievers and swigging pink liquids. Tired and stressed to the bone. People are knocking down my door to find the path to optimal health.

When I tell them that that path leads straight to the gut, they get skeptical. Especially if their bellies feel just fine.

But you don't have to have digestive complaints to be in the gutter. Yes, some illnesses cause belly symptoms like heartburn, constipation, diarrhea, and bloating. But there's now compelling evidence that ailments like food and environmental allergies, headaches, insomnia, skin irritations, low energy, and low libido—and many others—have a gut connection too. Heal the gut, and more often than not these maladies improve or are resolved entirely.

As you'll learn, healthy digestion depends on two things: a balance of friendly bacteria in the gut and a strong intestinal lining. Medical research backs up this claim. Consider these recent findings:

- A Harvard study found that high-fat, high-sugar diets may alter the gut's bacterial diversity, perhaps contributing to chronic illness.
- The composition of the microbial "stew" in your gut may influence your ability to absorb nutrients from food and, thus, your tendency to gain weight.
- In animal studies, gut bacteria influence brain chemistry and behavior. This finding could help people with gastrointestinal diseases, such as irritable bowel syndrome (IBS), that are associated with anxiety or depression.
- Some psychiatric disorders, including late onset autism, may be associated with abnormal bacterial content in the gut.
- The presence of the *Prevotella copri* bacterium in the gut is linked to the chronic inflammatory disorder rheumatoid arthritis, suggesting that this "gut bug" may play a part in this and perhaps other autoimmune diseases.
- People diagnosed with type 2 diabetes had lower levels of a microbe called butyrate, and produced more bacteria in general than nondiabetics, a Chinese study has found. This bacterium seems to have a protective role against this chronic disease.

The good news: Regardless of your current health, the 21-Day Belly Fix can "fire up" your gut, helping to rebalance your gut bacteria and strengthen or heal your intestinal lining.

A NATION IN THE GUTTER

Think of the rain gutters attached to buildings. Their main job is to control the flow of rainwater from the roof to the ground to prevent damage to the foundation through erosion. Clean your gutters regularly, and all will be well. Let them accumulate years of debris, and they can overflow, damaging the foundation and washing away the needed soil.

It's the same with your gut. If you periodically clean it out, you protect your foundation—your health. If you don't, it gets clogged with toxins.

Without a doubt, the main cause of clogged guts is our Western lifestyle. There's a steady diet of processed foods, bereft of nutrients but brimming with chemicals. A lack of exercise—we move our bodies little or not at all. (Or we exercise too much, which can be just as harmful to the gut.) Chemicals in the air and water. Stress. Frantic schedules that leave no time to prepare and enjoy fresh, wholesome food.

As with rain gutters, it's actually easier to unclog your gut periodically than to deal with the potential consequences of *not* doing so (even if it never seems convenient). Unfortunately, few take the time to clean either their gutters or their guts. The manufacturers of over-the-counter medications for digestive distress are making a fortune. But their products merely mask the symptoms of guts fouled with years of accumulated toxins and empty our wallets: Americans spend more than $100 billion a year on over-the-counter digestive aids—gas pills, antacids, and the like. The weight loss industry is also worth billions.

Digestive diseases, which include chronic constipation, gastroesophageal reflux disease (GERD), Crohn's disease, irritable bowel syndrome, and others—affect about 70 million Americans a year. It's estimated that up to 20 percent of Americans experience GERD symptoms—heartburn and reflux—once a week.

But those statistics are from 2004. A 2011 study published in the journal *Gut* suggests that GERD is on the rise. This one tracked more than thirty thousand people in Norway over eleven years. When it began, the prevalence of weekly heartburn and other symptoms of acid reflux was 11.6 percent. By the end, the prevalence had risen to 17.1 percent. That's a

47 percent increase! The potential cause of this stratospheric increase? Yet another epidemic you're likely familiar with: obesity.

The bottom line: Our guts are under siege. Chronic constipation, frequent diarrhea, an extra twenty pounds, constant heartburn, or abdominal pain that comes and goes are not symptoms to mask with pink liquids or pain relievers or diet books. They're warnings that the body is out of balance and on the path to disease.

Happily, more often than not, the gut forgives much—once it gets what it needs. But before you can feel good, lose weight, sleep soundly, have energy to burn, and actually resolve symptoms rather than cover them up with medications, you need to know what a healthy gut is. It's pretty simple. A healthy gut has two main characteristics: a balance of healthy bacteria and a strong intestinal lining. This was my guiding principle on my healing journey.

THE 21-DAY BELLY FIX BREAKTHROUGH

The 21-Day Belly Fix is the culmination of everything I've learned about the profound link between the gut and health. Blending ancient philosophies and techniques with the best of Western medicine and the latest in nutrition science, this 21-day program is designed to cleanse the belly of accumulated toxins. In just three weeks, it reprograms the digestive system, accelerates metabolism so you'll lose weight, and induces overall wellness.

Here's how this book is organized. Part 1 explores the workings of the digestive system and the interaction between it and other body systems. You'll learn more about that "second brain" too, as well as its profound effects on weight, mood, and sleep. Part 1 also reveals the major gut-depleters in your diet—sugar, fat, and refined grains—and expands on the keys to a maximized gut. And finally, you'll learn how to lose weight without dieting—the key to the plan.

Part 2 is the core, the food and lifestyle plan that is the 21-Day Belly Fix. On my regime, you'll nourish your body and gut with real, whole food—fruits and vegetables, yogurt and small amounts of fish and poul-

The 21-Day Belly Fix

Day 1	Day 2	Day 3	Day 4	Day 5	Day 6	Day 7
Get out of the Gutter			Plug Your Leaky Gut			Build Your Bacteria

Day 8	Day 9	Day 10	Day 11	Day 12	Day 13	Day 14
			Solve Your Food Puzzle			

Day 15	Day 16	Day 17	Day 18	Day 19	Day 20	Day 21
						BELLY FIXED!

try, my nutrient-laden Green Juice Blends and fermented foods that provide a natural source of healthy bacteria. Think of the 21-Day Belly Fix as a spa vacation for your gut. See the calendar above; it will take you through the entire protocol.

Part 3 explores the roles of stress and physical activity in gut health and offers simple, practical ways to stress less and move more each day. (Good news—intense exercise is bad for the gut, while slow, gentle exercise is healing.) I also offer alternative therapies from Chinese medicine and Ayurveda to add to your 21-Day Belly Fix if you desire.

The plan sounds simple; it is simple. But don't underestimate its power. I've seen it work wonders in thousands of my patients frustrated by their pain, excess weight, blue moods, and fatigue.

I put them on the 21-Day Belly Fix and schedule them for a three-week follow-up. When they return, even those who were the most doubtful are amazed. "Dr. Taz, I'm a new person!" exclaim some of them. And indeed, I can see that before I even examine them. They radiate health and energy. Their skin is clearer and smoother, they've lost weight, and they walk in beaming.

Once I do my exam and run some tests, the internal changes become evident too. Their levels of cholesterol and hemoglobin A1c (an indication of diabetes) have dropped. Their hormone balance has shifted. And the markers of inflammation (such as homocysteine) have improved dramatically.

The 21-Day Belly Fix has put thousands of my patients on the path to long-term health and vitality, as they feel fit and shed pounds. I'm confident that it can put you on the same path.

The 21-Day Belly Fix

one

The Fire in Your Belly

To understand how to lose weight with the 21-Day Belly Fix, you must first understand how the gut works so that you know what you're up against. And what you're up against is bad bacteria. As gross as it sounds, bacteria inhabit just about every part of your body, gut included. The tiny ecosystem in our bellies known as the gut microbiota contains tens of trillions of microorganisms. One third of your gut microbiota is common to most humans. Two thirds is specific to you, as unique as your fingerprint.

Under normal circumstances, this wide variety of gut bugs coexists peacefully, promoting proper digestive function, strong immunity, and overall vitality. But too many of the wrong bacteria, or not enough of the good ones, can have negative effects. This imbalance between the beneficial and harmful bacteria in the gut is known as *dysbiosis*—the opposite of symbiosis, which describes coexistence in a state of harmony.

Dysbiosis can make you feel nauseated, cause belly pain or bloating, or make you gassy (very gassy). Bowel movements change—you might have to "go" too much (diarrhea) or too little (constipation). You may also feel extremely tired; experience chronic pain from inflamed, aching joints; or feel mentally foggy. Sounds like fun, right?

The second characteristic of a healthy gut is a no-leak intestinal lining, the immune system's first line of defense. This lining looks like a net with very fine mesh. In a healthy gut, the holes are so tiny that only certain substances can pass through.

But if the lining is damaged, the holes get bigger. All sorts of undesirables—bacteria, viruses, yeast, undigested food particles—literally leak out of your small intestine into your bloodstream. The condition's formal name is "increased intestinal permeability," but it is more commonly known as leaky gut. Leaky gut can also lead to low-grade, body-wide inflammation and digestive issues, skin problems like psoriasis, and autoimmune diseases. People with leaky guts may also develop food sensitivities, because partially digested particles of protein and fat leaking through the intestinal wall into the bloodstream causes an allergic response. They may also be less able to absorb nutrients. And they may gain weight. With a leaky gut, the symptoms are all over the map. Digestive symptoms such as gas, bloating, and diarrhea may make life miserable. Your skin may break out in acne or other rashes. Your mood might change, and you may feel either depressed or anxious. You might develop seasonal allergies or even asthma.

I've treated thousands of people with leaky guts. Before they come through my door, they've seen doctor after doctor, taken test after test, and their symptoms are still a mystery, both to them and to the specialists they see. Tellingly, most Western-trained doctors don't believe leaky gut exists. It's practitioners who embrace alternative medicine systems who typically diagnose and treat it.

Here, let me touch briefly on the "second brain," housed in your gut. Called the enteric nervous system, the gut-brain is wired to the head-brain, and they're in constant communication. When all is well, the messages are quick updates. But if the gut is unhappy, it lets the brain know. A constant onslaught of negative messages from the gut can affect the nerve activity in the brain, leading to disturbances in mood and sleep.

But biology is only part of the 21-Day Belly Fix. The principles of Chinese medicine and Ayurveda are also very important to activating its full weight-loss potential.

YOUR DIGESTIVE FIRE

In your mind's eye, picture a roaring campfire. See the tongues of flame leap skyward. Feel the warmth of the flames on your face, in your bones. Hear the snap, crackle, and pop.

Now, imagine that campfire at dawn. The air is chill and damp. The fire is out, or nearly so. No light, no heat. Only scraps of charred wood, a thin wisp of smoke twisting in the air.

A fire burning up whatever is thrown into it, efficiently (good!) versus a pile of cold embers that lets whatever is tossed on top sit and rot (bad!). Those images suggest the two primary states of the digestive system in two ancient systems of healing, Chinese medicine and Ayurveda, the traditional medicine of India.

What is digestive fire? Each system approaches it from a slightly different angle. Chinese medicine (see page 10) focuses on diet. The stomach, it says, is a cooking pot; the spleen, which rules digestion, is the fire underneath the pot. Warmed by the spleen, the stomach cooks and breaks down what we eat. Eat well, and you'll feel well, because the food directly makes up our *qi*—our natural energy, a measure of our health and vitality.

Ayurveda, which originated in India almost three thousand years ago (see page 8), teaches that within each of us is a digestive fire that converts food to energy, and it's either in full blaze or a smoking pile of embers. A hot, bright blaze is the source of health, strength, nourishment, and energy. Yay! You must be eating a balanced diet. A smoky, smoldering fire weakens vitality, setting the stage for disease. Yikes. How many Dove Bars did you eat?

That rain-dampened campfire is the perfect way to picture chronic, low-grade inflammation in the body. Inflammation isn't always bad. It's part of the body's immune response, a natural reaction to injury and outside invaders. But there are two types of inflammation: acute and chronic.

The acute kind of inflammation is a protective response to irritation, trauma, or infection. Say you get a splinter in your finger. The injured tissue sends out signals to open blood vessels and allow fluids to move from the vessels to the injured tissue. The fluid carries blood cells and other substances that help fight infection and begin the repair process. The familiar signs of inflammation—redness, swelling, and pain—are caused by the increase in fluid around the injured area.

Chronic inflammation is another story. It's the damaging immune response caused by a variety of invaders including chemical toxins, food particles your gut can't digest, and even too much body fat. Like that rain-dampened campfire, chronic inflammation smokes and smolders continually. And over time, it wears down your immune system, paving the way for disease.

Maybe you already know that studies link chronic inflammation to cancer and cardiovascular disease. What you may not know is that it may play a role in Alzheimer's, celiac disease (CD), ulcerative colitis, Crohn's disease, the two most common types of inflammatory bowel disease (IBD), the debilitating autoimmune disease rheumatoid arthritis, and even obesity.

Both gut dysbiosis and a leaky gut trigger inflammation. Fortunately, the simple diet and lifestyle changes in the 21-Day Belly Fix help rebalance gut bacteria and seal a leaky intestinal lining, promoting good digestive health and quenching that smoldering, vitality-sapping inflammation. You can see how combining Western medicine with ancient medicine can benefit you.

AGNI AND AMA

In Ayurveda, the three doshas of vata, pitta, and kapha help form our unique constitutions, and they have a specific impact on bodily functions. Doshas are determined through medical history, exams, face readings, tongue and pulse readings, and personality assessments.

Furthermore, the doshas impact digestion, each in its unique way. That digestive fire I spoke of earlier? In Ayurveda, it's called *agni*. It's responsible for absorbing the nutrients the body needs while burning off waste products. When agni is strong, your metabolism hums, your body systems (digestive and others) work well individually and together, and you feel physically and mentally well, strong, and calm. A weak agni means an unbalanced body and mind. You feel sluggish, your mood takes a nosedive, your systems begin to malfunction, your skin and hair grow dull, and your metabolism slows considerably, leading to weight gain.

A weak agni is caused by a buildup of *ama*—undigested food that forms a toxic sludge within your digestive system. Ama is thought to lead to disease over time. I find it notable that a healthy mix of gut bacteria corresponds to agni, while a strong gut lining is one benefit of reducing ama.

Signs of ama include bad breath, a coated tongue, constipation, fatigue, and depression. (In Ayurveda, the inability to "digest" emotions—anger, sadness, guilt—can produce just as much ama as undigested food. Think of it as emotional sludge—toxic emotions that you can't eliminate.) To correct ama, Ayurveda recommends an individualized system that incorporates diet, herbal remedies, lifestyle modifications, and purification of digestion through fasting or detoxification.

The Chinese-medicine version of ama is known as "dampness" or "excessive phlegm." In these states, undigested food creates a sticky pudding-like mass in the body that causes "stagnation." In the language of mainstream medicine, stagnation is the inability of nutrients and blood to help other organ systems. Stagnation leads to "cold," which creates joint pain, constipation, hormone changes, and changes in mental health. Curing disease starts with correcting dampness or excess phlegm. The healing tools include herbs that relieve dampness, diet changes to reverse cold, and acupuncture to improve stagnation. All of these treatments strive to improve qi.

I love that these two ancient systems of medicine share the same goal: vibrant health, rather than symptom or disease management. It's a positive goal and a departure from the Western model of medicine.

Combining all the models is what makes the 21-Day Belly Fix work. The practice of integrative medicine is both art and science. This means that I rely on the diagnostic tools of Chinese and Ayurvedic medicine, based primarily on physical examination. But I confirm those diagnoses with conventional medical tests and add the latest breakthroughs in nutritional science to ancient healing diets.

Ayurveda 101

The word *Ayurveda* comes from two Sanskrit words: *ayur* (life) and *veda* (science or knowledge). Thus, this holistic system of medicine developed in India five thousand years ago is the science of life.

Mainstream medicine generally defines "good health" as the absence of disease. In Ayurveda, the definition is broader: a body, mind, and spirit in balance. The connection between balance and health trickled into mainstream medicine a few decades ago; Ayurveda identified it fifty centuries ago. This is the system of medicine Buddha used—high praise indeed.

Ayurvedic medicine centers on understanding a person's unique constitution, or *prakriti*. It teaches that we, and the world itself, are made up of five elements: earth, air, fire, water, and space. Each of these elements has certain qualities. For example, fire is hot and transformational, while earth is solid and stable.

Ayurveda places these elements into three main energies called *doshas*. There is *vata* (air and space), *pitta* (fire and water), and *kapha* (earth and water). Most of us are a combination of doshas. When you're treated by an Ayurvedic physician, his or her goal is to rebalance your body and mind and return you to your true constitution.

Here are characteristics of each dosha. Perhaps you will see yourself in one or two.

Pitta is derived from the Sanskrit word *pinj* ("to shine"). This dosha rules the small intestine and digestive and metabolic functions. Pitta-dominant people are typically aggressive achievers. They tend to have muscular builds, efficient metabolisms, and good appetites. Pitta is my dominant dosha, and I very much live up to this description!

In a figurative sense, pitta influences the ability to "digest" not just food but information, which we use to perceive the world. Pitta-dominant people are prone to nausea, vomiting, diarrhea, rashes, and anger. (Think about it— have you ever "acted rashly" in anger?) An excess of pitta can produce too much agni. To achieve balance, Ayurveda advises avoiding extreme heat and eating less spicy food.

Vata comes from the Sanskrit word *vayuu* ("that which moves"). Vata rules the colon and is seen as the force behind both pitta and kapha. Vata-dominant people are typically quick, alert, and restless. They may walk, talk, and think quickly, tend toward thinness, and be prone to nervousness or anxiety. Vata is believed to promote a balance between thought and emotion and to fuel creativity and clear comprehension.

Vata-dominant people tend to be susceptible to nerve disorders, insomnia, constipation, flatulence (oops), and arthritis. Unbalanced vata may show in the body as weight loss, constipation, hypertension, arthritis, weakness, and digestive issues. Most of my patients with anxiety are vata-dominant. Intense, adrenaline-pumping exercise like running or training for marathons can raise that dominance even higher. This is not a good situation, because an imbalance of vata can weaken agni.

To balance vata, Ayurvedic physicians advise staying calm (practicing stress management, in modern lingo), getting sufficient rest, and avoiding extreme temperatures.

Kapha is derived from the Sanskrit word *shlish* ("that which holds things together"). This dosha rules the stomach and governs immunity. Kapha-dominant people typically have significant physical and psychological strength and stability. However, they tend to overnurture and give away all their energy to others.

Kapha-dominant people are susceptible to lethargy, depression, allergies, and asthma. To maintain balance, they are advised to eat lightly, get frequent exercise, and avoid naps.

To identify a person's dosha (or doshas), an Ayurvedic physician examines their tongue, face, and eyes and takes their pulse. Then, he or she prescribes treatments and routines tailored to his or her prakriti and dosha. These might include diet and exercise recommendations, herbs, massage, and meditation.

It's fun to take one of those "What's your dosha?" quizzes on the Internet. But the complexities of Ayurveda can't be reduced to a quiz online, and only a trained practitioner can identify doshas accurately.

Chinese Medicine 101

I have studied many systems of medicine, but Chinese medicine may be my favorite. Maybe it's because this system has harnessed the healing power of nature in a complex and elegant system of protocols that has been used to enhance wellness and treat disease for over 2,500 years.

Chinese medicine is based on several core principles and concepts, including the one on which I founded my integrative practice: The health of mother and child are intimately connected. Here are other important concepts you need to know.

1. *Qi.* A vital "life energy" flows through us. This energy, *qi* (pronounced "chee"), travels along "pathways" in our bodies called meridians. If the flow of qi along these meridians becomes unbalanced or blocked, illness can occur. Causes of qi imbalance can involve lifestyle factors, such as poor diet or too little sleep, as well as stress, chronic illness, and excess medication intake.

2. *The Five Elements.* The Five Elements—earth, fire, wood, metal, and water—are aspects of qi, and they represent everything in the universe. They also explain how our bodies function and how disease changes that functioning. We shift through all of these elements over the course of our lives. However, one element typically dominates, and we can be "typed" by that element. Chinese medicine doctors use pulse and tongue and face reading to type their patients as well as to diagnose their health.

3. *Yin and yang.* All things, our bodies included, are made of two opposing but complementary forces: *yin* and *yang.* In Chinese medicine, hot versus cold (yin vs. yang) is vitally important. To maintain health and prevent illness, the body's balance of yin and yang must be maintained or restored.

4. As in Ayurvedic medicine, Chinese medicine treats the whole person— body, mind, and spirit. Its object is to help qi flow smoothly through the

body's meridians and to restore yin-yang balance. This balance creates vitality and good health and helps to prevent or treat disease.

5. Chinese medicine doctors use a variety of methods. These include:

    1. *Diet.* Balancing our consumption of foods that are "cold" (yin) and "hot" (yang) helps to balance the flow of qi. "Cold" and "hot" refer not to the temperature of these foods but to their effects on the body. You eat the proper balance of "cold" and "hot" foods for you.

    2. *Chinese herbal medicine.* The Chinese *Materia Medica*, a pharmacological reference book, describes thousands of medicinal substances, mostly plant leaves, roots, stems, flowers, and seeds. Often, practitioners combine them in formulas and prescribe them in teas, capsules, liquid extracts, and powders. Many of my patients bring their customized herbal medicines from their Chinese medicine practitioners to my office—bags of crushed, dried white peony petals or spicy-sweet powdered ginger root from which they make tea or soup, bottles of herbal blends steeped in alcohol (called tinctures), syrups made from wood bark, dandelion leaves, milk thistle flowers.

    3. *Acupuncture.* The body's meridians are dotted with specific points through which qi can be accessed. Inserting thin, solid, metal needles at these points releases qi, freeing it to flow throughout the body. As a licensed acupuncturist, I have used this technique to treat all kinds of conditions, including abdominal pain and IBS.

    4. *Acupressure.* An alternative to acupuncture, acupressure also moves qi. Practitioners apply direct pressure to points along the body's meridians using their hands or fingers or tape magnets, seeds, or even rocks over acupuncture points. I use acupressure to help my patients manage stress, quell the nausea of pregnancy, quit smoking, or manage overeating.

5. *T'ai chi.* This ancient Chinese system of exercise combines dance-like movements with breathing and relaxation. The specific movements are considered to move qi. I often recommend t'ai chi to older patients, patients who are not ready for moderate-intensity workouts but who would benefit from exercise.

If you're interested in experiencing Chinese medicine for yourself, I recommend finding a practitioner who is licensed, certified, and experienced. The United States accredits schools in Chinese medicine, so search for a practitioner certified by an accredited school and licensed by your state.

Also, as ancient Chinese and Ayurvedic healers did, I view each patient as unique—a fusion of inborn traits and external choices and habits that, together, affect their health. These unique qualities suggest the appropriate treatments. In some patients, symptoms of a dosha imbalance are very apparent. In others, it's the symptoms of blocked qi, dampness, or heat that leap out at me. Sometimes, I use acupuncture, acupressure, or Chinese herbs to return the body to balance. And sometimes, it's the healing foods of Ayurveda (kitchari, ghee, ginger) or the Ayurvedic practices of yoga and abdominal massage that bring relief.

You, too, are unique. The strength of the 21-Day Belly Fix program is that it's designed around treatments that are healing for the majority of my patients. Used in combination, each treatment—diet, herbs, supplements, exercise, stress management—is far more powerful than it is in isolation. Together, they return the body to balance, and balance is the 21-Day Belly Fix's overriding goal.

The key to a 21-Day Belly Fix success is identifying your unique food story, understanding your dosha and your Chinese meridian diagnosis, rebuilding your gut bacteria, and identifying your core gut issues. In our practice, we use Chinese medicine pulse and tongue readings, meridian analysis, Ayurvedic pulse readings, and conventional patient histories and physical exams, along with measuring pH and running blood tests to help nail the diagnosis. In this book, you benefit from the combined wisdom of thousands of patients seen in my practice and successfully treated using this approach.

HOW BADLY DO YOU NEED A 21-DAY BELLY FIX?

Based on core principles of nutrition, Chinese medicine, Ayurveda, and Western medicine, this simple yes-or-no quiz can help you gauge your level of ama. Circle the response that best describes you, awarding yourself one point for every yes answer and zero points for a no response. The more yeses you have, the higher the likelihood that you're in the gutter.

Face

In Chinese and Ayurvedic medicine, your face reveals your health. Ama, dampness, and stagnation show up on your face—and often, cosmetics can't hide them.

1. You have dark circles under your eyes. Y   N
2. You have rashes that are red and irritated (includes acne, eczema, rosacea, or any red irritation). Y   N
3. Your face is puffy or swollen. Y   N
4. Your tongue has a white or yellow coating. Y   N
5. Your skin color is/has been described as pale or dull. Y   N

Energy Level

Are you often fatigued and mentally foggy? Do you joke about "carb comas"? The health of your gut and the health of your diet can dramatically affect your energy levels. If you've ever done a detoxification diet, you know that it makes your energy skyrocket. Just a few days into your 21-Day Belly Fix, your energy level will soar.

6. You are tired after you eat. Y   N
7. You often suffer from "brain fog." Y   N
8. You get sick more than four times per year. Y   N

Digestive Symptoms

I am always surprised how many of my patients dismiss these. Perhaps it's because they have come to depend on over-the-counter medications to relieve them. The 21-Day Belly Fix gets to the root of these symptoms, healing them gently but for good.

9. You do not have a bowel movement every day. Y   N
10. You have abdominal pain more than twice a month. Y   N
11. You experience gas or bloating after a meal. Y   N
12. You have loose, unformed stools three or more times per week. Y   N
13. Your stools float, rather than sink to the bottom of the toilet. Y   N

Diagnosed Health Conditions

Circle the condition(s) you have been diagnosed with. They may be connected to microbial imbalances in your gut or a leaky intestinal lining, even if your symptoms don't affect your belly.

14. Chronic allergies or asthma Y   N
15. Hormone imbalances Y   N
16. Infertility Y   N
17. Anxiety or depression Y   N
18. Chronic vitamin B_{12} or iron deficiency Y   N

Family History

Circle the condition(s) that run in your family. There's good evidence that genetic predisposition is one factor in the conditions listed below. For example, relatives of people who have IBD have at least a tenfold increased risk for the disease.

19. Colon or breast cancer Y   N
20. Inflammatory bowel disease (IBD) Y   N
21. Irritable bowel syndrome (IBS) Y   N

Medications

Many of my patients come to me believing that medications are the answer—but they can cause more problems than they solve. Often, I can resolve the root of their ailments with simple, natural treatments.

22. You use ibuprofen or other pain relievers more than 3 times per week. Y   N
23. You use antacids or reflux medications more than 3 times per week. Y   N

Weight

When there's a doughnut shop or fast-food restaurant on every corner, it's not hard to gain weight. But an imbalanced gut may add fuel to our obesogenic environment. Evidence suggests that the gut microbiota may play a role in the development of obesity and that eating a healthy diet encourages microbes associated with leanness to become incorporated into the gut.

24. I continue to gain weight despite positive lifestyle changes. Y   N
25. I tend to lose weight or have a hard time keeping it on. Y   N

Portrait of a Man in the Gutter

The seventy-two-year-old sitting across from me was a character—sharp and witty, with a loud voice and a deep belly laugh. But this seemingly healthy and vibrant man hadn't come to entertain me. He was battling Stage IV colon cancer. Having endured three rounds of chemotherapy, he wanted to know whether I could do anything more for him.

He'd been raised in India, with an Ayurvedic physician in the house. "He'd look at our tongues and face to check our digestion," he recalled. "The minute he thought it was off, we had to fast, drinking only water for a day. The next day, he'd make us kitchari, a dish made of lentils and rice thought in Ayurveda to be easily digestible."

"I was raised this way. I ate this way. Then, at twenty-five, I came to the United States and started to eat whatever I wanted—pizza, sweets, chips." He paused, closing his eyes briefly. "And now, here I sit, with colon cancer."

His tale saddened me. It also gave me the chills. In him I saw my husband, Vik, thirty years in the future. My patient hailed from the same region of India as he did. They had similar personalities. And both ate poor diets.

Spooked, I sent him from my office to Vik's, which is right across the street. I wanted him to tell my husband about the consequences of his lifetime of poor food choices and what they had now cost him. I did not want this lovely man's fate to become his.

This man was my husband's wake-up call. He must have heard it loud and clear, because, these days, I see more vegetables on his plate and less ice cream in his bowl. Unlike my patient, Vik has time to get out of the gutter and live a long life. And you do too.

Scoring

0-8 POINTS: Outstanding! Your agni is in full blaze (something I rarely see in first-time patients). To keep your digestive fire burning hot and bright, follow the 21-Day Belly Fix twice a year.

9-16 POINTS: Wake-up call! You may feel fine now, but at some point your digestive fire will begin to sputter and smoke. The resulting cold or dampness throughout your body will rob you of your vitality and increase your risk of disease. The 21-Day Belly Fix can reverse this trend—if you start now.

17-25 POINTS: You may be struggling with a multitude of symptoms, which may or may not be causing digestive issues. But it's never too late to get out of the gutter! Schedule an appointment with your doctor. Bring this book and get the green light to follow the 21-Day Belly Fix. Coupled with a doctor's care, this program can help rebalance your gut bacteria, strengthen your intestinal lining, and clean your gut of its accumulated toxins, which are likely at the root of your symptoms.

two

The "Guts" of Your Gut

Weak agni. Too much ama. A gut that leaks. Twenty extra pounds around your middle. If you've got 'em, you need a 21-Day Belly Fix. But as you'll see, your digestive system goes way, *way* beyond your stomach.

A few years back, my family took a vacation to the Cayman Islands. My sweet children, then toddlers, were captivated by the ocean—how it changed color from hour to hour, the ceaseless churn of the waves. One day, eager to see the life that flourished beneath the surface of the water, we climbed into a submarine for a tour.

Until this point, my children had seen only the waves that extended for as far as their eyes could see. Once underwater, they were equally amazed by the world that lay beneath the surface—the coral reefs and underwater vegetation, the vibrant and varied species of fish. As I write this chapter, I think back to that day. Like the ocean, the digestive system and its work go way beyond what we see or think we know.

The digestive organs are exquisitely designed, their work enormously complicated. They are of two types, hollow and solid. The "hollow" organs are the mouth, esophagus, stomach, and small intestine, and they are

Your Gut: More Than a "Food Tube"

Oceans provide us with food and relaxation. We want them resilient to harmful algae blooms, oil spills, and toxic chemicals. While a healthy ocean can withstand such calamities, constant stressors eventually can undermine its ability to recover.

It's the same with your digestive system. A junk-food diet, no exercise, and constant worry disrupt the balance it needs to function at its peak. Its friendly bacteria can be overrun by bad bugs. Its intestinal wall, once sealed up tight, can develop holes, which increases its vulnerability to invaders. As you'll recall, a weak agni means a body and mind out of balance. And it's ama—undigested food that coats your digestive system with toxic sludge—that's the main cause of this unhealthy disharmony.

Your GI tract controls digestion and the absorption of food and nutrients and ultimately determines your nutritional status. However, your digestive system is more than your GI tract. There are three other parts, each critical to proper digestion and vibrant health.

The gut immune system. Do you get over one cold, only to get sick again right away? Or battle chronic allergies no matter what time of year it is? Chances are you need a 21-Day Belly Fix. Seventy percent of your body's immune system is located in the gut, just under the surface of the gut lining. This lining is your body's first line of defense against invaders.

It's like this. Your skin is a physical barrier between the "inner you" and the toxic world "out here." When your skin is broken, as it is when you have a cut, invaders can use that break to enter your body and get into your bloodstream.

Your gut lining has a "skin," too. When intact, invaders can't sneak inside you and enter your bloodstream. But if this "inner skin" is broken, they can enter the breach and make you sick. Lifestyle choices, particularly diet, can help you protect this skin within or weaken it.

The bugs in your gut. There's much exciting research that connects gut microbiology to the prevention of disease. You can thank the huge colony of "good" bacteria in your gut, which plays a vital role in a healthy immune system. Among their many roles, these friendly bacteria:

- reduce inflammation in the gut;
- help stimulate the immune system's production of white blood cells, which defend against disease;
- rev up metabolism;
- produce acids that help break food down into easily digestible particles; and
- help break down certain B vitamins, which help your body get or make energy from food, and vitamin K, which plays a major role in the ability of the blood to clot.

The brain in your gut. It's true! This "second brain" makes and processes critical chemicals and hormones essential to health and proper digestion. The gut-brain and head-brain "talk" all the time, and when one is unhappy, the other hears about it. I'll discuss this "belly brain" in the next chapter. For now, let's focus on the phases of digestion—from the "surface" stages to the "deep-sea" points—and how a healthy GI tract works in perfect harmony with its other parts.

joined together by the long, snake-like tube of your gastrointestinal tract (GI tract). The "solid" organs are the liver, pancreas, and gallbladder. All work together to turn a meal into nutrients that your body's cells can use for energy and repair.

In a complex and synchronized process, the digestive system, aided by the endocrine, immune, and nervous systems, processes every nibble, morsel, and Pepperidge Farm Mint Milano you swallow each day. Its organs squirt it with enzymes that break it down into ever-smaller molecules. Churn it first into a nutrient-dense paste and then a liquid. Extract and absorb its nutrients. It's a bit like an action movie: Every moment, "invaders"—incompletely digested proteins and fats, environmental chemicals, bacteria that cause illness, toxic byproducts of hormone production, parasites—are targeted, attacked, and neutralized.

Once the digestive system has wrung every nutrient from your meal, only the indigestible parts remain. But even that waste is precious. It feeds the friendly bacteria in your large intestine, or colon. To return the favor, these "good" bacteria promote proper and soul-satisfying elimination. (Yes, we're talking about poop, people!)

There are four phases of digestion, each with specific processes that directly affect your health. To extend my ocean metaphor, the first two can be viewed as "surface" phases; the latter two are "deep-sea" phases, where the complex work of digestion, nutrient absorption, and immune function primarily are conducted. The food we eat? That's the submarine. On the surface, all you see—and taste—is a delightful meal. But with your first swallow, the "surface phase" of digestion ends and the "underworld" takes over.

Ready to take a deep dive? Hold your breath . . .

DIGESTION'S "SURFACE" PHASES

(1) The Cephalic Phase: The Eyes Eat First

Imagine a thin-crust pizza bubbling with mozzarella and dotted with salty, chewy pepperoni. Can you taste it? Your brain can, and so can your gut, before you've even taken the first luscious bite.

The Japanese say "the eyes eat first," and it's true—this first phase of digestion is all in your head. This "mind-centered" phase preps your digestive organs for action. Thinking about food triggers saliva and digestive juices and enzymes—which will be needed once food hits your stomach—and increases blood flow to your digestive organs.

But that's a textbook description. How well this phase goes depends on whether your body and mind are chilled out or overloaded on teeth-grinding, boss-blaming, desk-rattling stress. And that depends on a particular part of your nervous system: the autonomic nervous system.

There are three branches of the autonomic nervous system, and each plays a role in how you're digesting that cookie. The *sympathetic nervous system* governs the body's stress response, which prepares the body to fight a threat or flee from it. That's why the stress response is often called "fight or flight"! Under severe stress, digestion slows or shuts down completely. (When your gut-brain and head-brain perceive danger, digesting your late-night snack is pretty far down on their to-do list.) If the stress is acute enough, you might feel like you're about to lose your lunch, or even (to put it impolitely) sh*t yourself. We've all been there, and it's no laughing matter, unless you count the people laughing at you.

By contrast, the *parasympathetic nervous system* regulates "rest and digest" functions. It's the state associated with the relaxation response. When activated, it promotes digestion. It stands to reason, then, that you want to eat in a blissed-out, ahhhhh state.

Of course, this doesn't happen very often. Our everyday worries can have a powerful—and unhealthy—effect on the gut. We may be aware that stress is a constant in our lives but discount its effect on our health and digestion. The reality is, the consequences of chronic stress, which include reduced production of stomach acid and reduced absorption of nutrients, reverberate through each phase of digestion. For example, stress also reduces *motility,* or the contraction of the muscles in the digestive tract. As a result, food just sits in your stomach, which can cause indigestion, gas, and bloating.

Because your eyes eat first, it's important to eat only when you are in a relaxed state. Take just twenty minutes to sit down to eat a meal, rather than choke it down in the car or while you pay bills online (remember what happened to me, when I ate and ran in the ER?). If you love to cook, make the time—as you chop herbs and inhale fragrant aromas, your digestive juices will start to flow. Then sit down at the table and savor it, happily and peacefully.

Diet and weight management experts frequently mention "our relationship with food," yet we rarely give food the time and attention we lavish on our significant other or best friend. Choose each meal the way you'd choose a lover. Give mealtime your full attention. Don't gobble your food—romance it! Your gut will thank you. When you're forced to eat and run, at least perform a quick relaxation exercise to activate the rest-and-digest response, such as the 1:4:7 breath that I myself use, which is explained in chapter 12. Such small steps can help promote digestion and a happier belly.

(2) The Esophageal Phase: The Gateway to GERD

When you chew and swallow a bite of food, it passes into your esophagus, the tube that connects the throat and the stomach. But although lubricated by saliva, that bite doesn't just slide down the esophagus. This tube has muscles, and those muscles *push*. You don't think it's true now, but pay attention next time you're eating and you can almost feel it.

When muscles in the esophagus (and elsewhere in the digestive tract) contract in a synchronized way to move food from organ to organ, it's called peristalsis. Think of waves breaking on the shore, and you get an idea of peristalsis—a series of rhythmic, wave-like contractions that move food from esophagus to stomach, stomach to small intestine, small intestine to colon.

When your esophagus works properly, you don't give it much thought unless you try to swallow something too large, too hot, or too cold. The wild card? A small ring of muscle at the end of the esophagus called the lower esophageal sphincter (LES), which separates the esophagus from the stomach.

When you swallow, the LES opens, or relaxes, so that chewed food can enter the stomach. Once food is in the stomach, it closes, which prevents food and acid from washing up from the stomach ("refluxing") and back into the esophagus. But if the LES doesn't close well, acid from the stomach can splash upward, or "reflux," and burn the moist, soft lining of the esophagus. This is called reflux, or gastroesophageal reflux disease (GERD).

As you learned in chapter 1, GERD is an overlooked epidemic. If you ignore this critical phase of digestion, you risk sowing the seeds of this uncomfortable and sometimes dangerous condition. Classic signs of

What the Heck Is pH?

Way back in your high school chemistry class, you probably learned about pH, short for "potential hydrogen." In basic terms, pH measures how acidic or alkaline a liquid is. It is measured on a scale of 0 to 14. The lower the pH, the more acidic the liquid; the higher the pH, the more alkaline the liquid. When a liquid is neither acid nor alkaline, it has a pH of 7, which is neutral. Water is "pH neutral."

Because our bodies are 70 percent water, pH is used to describe the acidity or alkalinity of our bodies. The overall pH of a healthy body is neutral, and it strives to keep that balance. By contrast, the pH of a healthy belly is around 1–3 when empty, rising to 4–5 after a meal.

That's a pretty acidic environment, and stomach acid itself is a blistering brew, with a pH of about 0.8–1.0. That's as strong as battery acid! But this acidity suits the stomach just fine.

As you can see, digestive pH, which *should* be acidic, differs from overall body pH, which should *not* be acidic. "Over-acidity" in the body creates an unbalanced internal environment that promotes disease. And "under-acidity" in the stomach can slow digestion, which creates a paradise for bad bacteria that can make you sick and increase the risk of disease. In my practice, we test the pH of patients' saliva or urine to determine overall pH. A pH under 6.8 suggests that the body is too acidic and that the stomach is not acidic enough.

GERD include heartburn two or more times a week, a sour taste in the mouth, burning in the throat, and chest pain. "Silent" symptoms include a dry cough, a hoarse voice, difficulty swallowing, or the feeling of a lump in the throat. Either way, it's important to heal the condition rather than just mask the symptoms with the pink stuff. On this program, you can.

DIGESTION'S "DEEP-SEA" PHASES

(3) The Gastric Phase: The "pH Test" of Digestion

Think of digestion, and you think stomach. And this organ—shaped like a crescent roll—certainly is the headliner of this phase, which starts the moment food from the esophagus hits it. But proper pH balance, both in the body and the stomach, also plays a critical role. To put it simply, the body needs the right balance of acids and non-acids (alkalis) in its tissues, blood, saliva, and urine to be healthy. That's what pH levels measure— this balance of acids and alkalis.

The pH of your stomach is determined by the quality and quantity of your *gastric juice,* a mix of hydrochloric acid, digestive enzymes, and mucus. Further, for gastric juice to do its important work, your stomach must have the proper pH balance.

Many of my patients have read that a healthy body has an alkaline pH (or a pH of greater than 6.8 when measured in the urine or saliva). So they think that the stomach's pH should be alkaline too. Not true! A healthy stomach is highly acidic. The acid is what begins the digestive process. When acid supplies are low, the GI system doesn't extract the right nutrients from food and has to work much harder to process the food. And although just one drop of stomach acid would eat through your skin (think of the alien in *Alien*), in the stomach it's just fine—mucus protects its lining from the blistering brew.

Another problem in this phase: eating too much. When the stomach's smooth muscles begin peristalsis, churning food and gastric juice like a washing machine, this organ needs room to *work.* If it's full to the brim, peristalsis slows down, and your huge meal . . . just . . . sits . . . for longer than it should. This is called *gastroparesis,* or delayed stomach emptying. Your stomach will return this mistreatment with gas, bloating, and stomach pain. A meal that contains too much fat, or too much of the wrong kind of fat, also delays stomach emptying and can result in the same symptoms. On the other hand, the healthy fats included in the 21-Day

Belly Fix stimulate gut motility, aid in elimination and detoxification, and help the right balance of gut bugs.

Overeating can also build pressure in your stomach. This can pop open the LES, causing the misery of heartburn. (I always advise my patients to pretend they're in Europe, where portion sizes are small and mealtimes relaxed. Europeans really know how to pamper their digestive systems. French women don't get fat, right?)

Low stomach acid can muck up this phase, too. It can slow digestion way down—and that slowdown can breed trouble in the gut in the form of bad bugs. The stomach wants to keep that pulpy mess of partly digested food and gastric juices—called chyme—until it reaches the proper pH level. Without adequate amounts of stomach acid, it sits in the stomach for a longer period, and the nutrients cannot be broken down properly. This promotes the growth of harmful bacteria in the small intestine, which can lead to *small intestinal bacterial overgrowth* (SIBO). This condition is associated with a wide variety of disorders and diseases, from chronic diarrhea and migraines to hypothyroidism, IBS, and fibromyalgia.

If you suffer chronic heartburn or GERD, there's a good chance that your stomach isn't making too much acid but too *little*. This is especially true if you're in middle age (when gastric acid secretion typically declines) or take antacids or medications that suppress acid production (which reduce the little acid your stomach does produce). If your stomach acid is low, *any* amount that refluxes into your esophagus can cause heartburn or silent symptoms.

Often, medications are short-term fixes rather than long-term solutions. Many of my patients are delighted to find out that it's the 21-Day Belly Fix program, rather than a long list of medications, that corrects low stomach acid and the accompanying heartburn or reflux and prevents the bacterial overgrowth that can lead to SIBO.

When Food Attacks, Suspect a Leaky Gut

Leaky gut is a prime suspect behind food *allergy* and food *intolerance*. Both can cause vomiting, diarrhea, or abdominal cramps and pain. But there's a big difference between the two: an immune response, or a lack of one.

In a food allergy, the immune system lashes out at something it shouldn't: a protein in an otherwise healthy food. When the protein enters the digestive system, an antibody called immunoglobulin E (IgE) is produced. In minutes or even seconds, IgE triggers an allergic response that can range from mild to severe. Reactions can take the form of nausea, vomiting, cramps, or diarrhea. They can also affect the skin (hives or swelling of the lips, face, or throat) or respiratory system. In severe cases, the life-threatening allergic reaction of anaphylaxis can occur. In adults, the foods that most often trigger allergic reactions include fish, shellfish, peanuts, and tree nuts, such as walnuts. (In children, the foods are slightly different: eggs, milk, peanuts, tree nuts, soy, and wheat.)

An intolerance to a certain food—to the lactose found in cow's milk or to the gluten in wheat, oats, barley, and rye—is more common than food allergy. An intolerance doesn't trigger an immune response and is not life-threatening, as a food allergy can be. This time, a different immunoglobulin is involved: IgG, which may take hours or even days to produce many of the same symptoms as food allergy.

But that doesn't mean food intolerance is not serious, even though most mainstream physicians downplay the possibility that the vague symptoms it can produce—such as brain fog, moodiness, and sleep problems—might be diet-related. Food intolerances begin as a slow decline in health, gradually chipping away at the immune system and impairing the gut lining's ability to absorb nutrients. Stress, illness, or a particular medication produces a "tipping point," and the slow decline becomes full-blown inflammation. That's when people come to me with gut-wrenching digestive symptoms as well as migraines, eczema, and sinusitis. Once you begin the

21-Day Belly Fix, you'll pinpoint the problem foods for you—the ones you should eat infrequently, if at all. Once you zero in on and eliminate them, those conditions improve and often vanish entirely.

(4) The Intestinal Phase: Absorption, Absorption, Absorption

If all goes well in this phase, nutrients are absorbed and pass through the intestinal walls and into the bloodstream, where they nourish every cell in your body. But if it goes wrong . . . welcome to Atlanta! Because sadly, that means I gain another patient.

This phase begins when the stomach empties your now liquefied meal into your small intestine. Imagine a twenty-foot garden hose, one inch in diameter, coiled up inside your abdominal cavity. That's the small intestine, which processes about 2.5 gallons of food, liquids, and waste a day.

The intestinal lining is packed with hair-like projections called *villi*. When I say packed, I mean it: One square inch of small intestine contains about twenty thousand villi. It's these tiny, hairlike projections that allow nutrients from food to be absorbed into the bloodstream.

But if the villi are damaged, problems ensue. It's said that we are what we eat, but that's not strictly true. You can eat a healthy diet but be unable to absorb its nutrients. The situation is akin to placing a call when your cell phone has no bars: Nothing gets through. If things go awry in this phase, you can eat clean, take supplements—and still end up malnourished.

This is what happens when people with celiac disease ingest gluten. Their immune systems mount a ferocious response to that protein that damages the villi, reducing their ability to soak up nutrients. The other symptoms of CD are equally serious—abdominal pain, cramps, nausea, vomiting and diarrhea, bloating, moodiness, and mental fogginess.

However, it's possible to feel perfectly well and *still* be unable to absorb the nutrients from food. Years of the wrong foods, the wrong digestive pH, and constant stress can *also* block absorption of nutrients, leading to too much ama and weak agni.

Even if the villi function well, absorbed nutrients still have to pass through the intestinal wall and into the bloodstream. But invaders are lurking. Just one layer of cells separates your intestinal wall from the outside world—a hostile world, rife with undigested food particles and various microbes, molecules, and toxins. This lining must let nutrients pass into the bloodstream as it keeps invaders out. The gut immune system coordinates the process of detoxification, and there is no margin for error.

LEAKY GUT: A BREACH OF SECURITY

In chapter 1, you learned that leaky gut is the result of undesirable molecules and microorganisms leaking through the intestinal wall into the bloodstream. This leakage sets the stage for digestive symptoms, food allergy and intolerance, and autoimmune diseases. While simple, natural treatments can help solve this problem, it's helpful to understand what's going on first.

As mentioned, the intestinal lining is the immune system's first line of defense. The outer layers of intestinal cells are connected by structures called tight junctions. Just like filling up nail holes in a wall with spackle, tight junctions fill in the spaces between cells. In a healthy gut, the cells of the intestinal wall are tightly packed, and the tight junctures between these cells are sound. No holes. No gaps. The fine mesh of a strong intestinal lining allows nutrients to enter the bloodstream and to repel invaders.

With a leaky gut, either the cells of the intestinal wall are damaged or the tight junctions loosen. Both scenarios can produce larger holes or gaps that allow invaders to pass directly into the bloodstream. Responding to this breach in security, the gut immune system swings into action, releasing white blood cells to attack the invaders.

A poor diet, an imbalanced gut microbiota, environmental toxins, stress, and large amounts of non-steroidal anti-inflammatory drugs (NSAIDs) such as aspirin and ibuprofen can lead to gut leakiness and inflammation. The gut gets locked into an endless cycle. Leaky gut leads to inflammation; inflammation leads to disease. This unhealthy cycle creates body-wide (systemic) inflammation, the igniting factor for *all* the diseases of modern civilization, including celiac disease, type 2 diabetes, cancer, heart disease, ADHD, and autism. Which disease may develop depends on an individual's unique genetic predisposition.

No doubt you've heard a lot about celiac disease in the past few years. Perhaps you've even been diagnosed with it after months (or years!) of abdominal bloating and pain, diarrhea, or constipation. Leaky gut may be the culprit. In fact, almost every autoimmune disease begins with a leaky gut. And what else? Yes, weight gain.

I often joke that I run a rheumatology clinic, since so many of my patients seek answers to a particular autoimmune disease, from vitiligo to ulcerative colitis. The cause varies from patient to patient—for one it's a food intolerance, for another low stomach acid. But the treatment is always the same: a 21-Day Belly Fix. What will help plug a leaky gut: controlling inflammation by eating the right foods for you and taking the right blend of amino acids (the building blocks of protein) and supplements such as glutamine, aloe vera juice, and digestive enzymes.

THE COLON: THE END OF THE LINE

The end of the digestive process heralds the beginning of a critical post-digestive phase: pooping. The importance of at least one bulky, satisfying bowel movement a day cannot be overstated—it's an essential part of digestive health. So although it's not strictly part of the digestive system, your colon plays a critical role in your digestive health.

After your small intestine has absorbed the nutrients from your meal and your liver has processed them, all that's left of your once-delicious meal is the stuff that can't be digested, mostly fiber and water. Peristalsis in the small intestine moves those indigestible remains to your colon. This long muscular tube, four to six feet long, absorbs water and electrolytes (such as sodium and potassium) from food. Just as important: The colon compacts solid waste so that the body can eliminate it.

Ayurvedic and Chinese medicine recognized thousands of years ago that undigested material that sits in the colon produced toxins and led to disease. If you told me that you moved your bowels only a few times a week, I'd be concerned, because constipation increases ama.

When the remains of your meal hit your colon, the enormous colony of bacteria in your colon puts on the feed bag. Good gut bugs *love* fiber. The healthier your diet, the more often nature calls, and the more ama you eliminate from your body.

Ideally, most gut bacteria stays in your colon. And in an ideal world in which everyone ate a wide variety of plant-based foods and took medications sparingly, that's where they'd stay. A clean diet and healthy lifestyle help invite the right mix of bacteria, parasites, and yeast into the colon, which leads to happy and harmonious gut microbiology.

If the colon lacks this diversity, the waste just sits there, and you develop constipation, a prime cause of ama. In Ayurvedic medicine, this ama creates digestive heat. This kicks off the pattern of heat-based illnesses, including eczema, acne, and hair loss. Things get worse if bugs move into your small intestine. That's when an overgrowth of yeast, an overgrowth of bacteria, or infections from parasites can result in infection, SIBO, and candida.

It doesn't have to be this way. In the coming chapters, you'll learn to use food, supplements, and other natural treatments to make your body a welcoming host. For example, fermented foods (such as coconut milk yogurt, sauerkraut, tempeh, and miso) are a natural source of healthy bacteria, and onions, dandelion greens, and chicory are *prebiotics,* which serve as food for healthy gut bugs.

WHEN THE GUT GOES WRONG

It's beyond the scope of this book to describe in detail specific medical conditions associated with gut dysfunction. However, the following charts will give you a sense of the strong link between digestive and overall health, what can happen when the gut goes wrong, and conventional versus integrative treatment options for those conditions. They also link Ayurvedic and Chinese medicine thought with the diseases of today.

Chart 1 displays four major digestive diseases and their symptoms as well as other diseases related to them. Chart 2 displays other symptoms

Chart 1

Disease	Systemic Symptoms/Illnesses	Conventional Treatment
Celiac Disease	Type 1 diabetes	Gluten avoidance, anti-inflammatory medications like prednisone, immunosuppressants (6-mercaptopurine, methotrexate), thyroid medications (Synthroid), anti-epileptic drugs, antidepressants or anti-anxiety medications (Wellbutrin, Lexapro, Prozac), iron replacement (synthetic Fe), insulin replacement
	Autoimmune thyroid disease	
	Autoimmune liver disease	
	Rheumatoid arthritis	
	Addison's disease, a condition in which the glands that produce critical hormones are damaged	
	Sjögren's syndrome, a condition in which the glands that produce tears and saliva are destroyed	
	Unexplained iron-deficiency anemia	
	Fatigue	
	Bone or joint pain	
	Arthritis	
	Bone loss or osteoporosis	
	Depression or anxiety	
	Tingling numbness in the hands and feet	
	Seizures	
	Missed menstrual periods	
	Infertility or recurrent miscarriage	
	Canker sores inside the mouth	
	An itchy skin rash called dermatitis herpetiformis	
GERD	Dry, chronic cough	Proton pump inhibitors (Prilosec), acid blockers (Zantac)
	Sleep disturbances	
	Wheezing	
	Asthma	
	Recurrent pneumonia	
	Nausea/vomiting	
	Sore throat, hoarseness, or laryngitis	
	Difficult or painful swallowing	
	Pain in the chest or the upper part of the abdomen	
	Dental erosion and bad breath	
IBD	Arthritis and joint pain	Steroids (prednisone, Canasa), immunosuppressants, biologics (Humira, Remicade)
	Eye disorders (uveitis, iritis)	
	Mouth ulcers (aphthous stomatitis)	
	Skin lesions (pyoderma gangrenosum, erythema nodosum)	
IBS	Chronic fatigue syndrome	Dietary fiber, antispasmodics (Bentyl, Levsin), antidiarrheal agents (loperamide), antidepressants/anti-anxiety medications (citalopram, Lexapro)
	Chronic pelvic pain	
	Problems or symptoms of the chewing muscles and joints that connect the lower jaw to the skull	
	Depression or anxiety	
	Restless leg syndrome	
	Somatoform disorders—chronic pain or other symptoms with no physical cause that are thought to be due to psychological problems	

Integrative Medicine Diagnosis	Integrative Treatment
Spleen qi deficiency, spleen-pancreas disharmony, liver-kidney disharmony, pitta/vata imbalance, leaky gut (intestinal dysbiosis), SIBO, candida	Diet: gluten avoidance; increase iron-rich foods, especially heme iron in red meat, chicken, and mutton, a favorite in Chinese medicine; foods that improve gut immunology—fermented foods; little or minimal sugar. Supplements: glutamine to rebuild gut lining, probiotics, colostrum (adds immunoglobulins to GI system), supplemental heme iron (liver derived)
Rebellious liver qi, spleen qi deficiency, food allergies, food intolerances, leaky gut	Diet: anti-inflammatory, removal of alcohol and caffeine. Supplements: glutamine, slippery elm and digestive enzymes, probiotics
Spleen qi deficiency, spleen-kidney disharmony, liver-kidney disharmony, pitta/vata imbalance, leaky gut (intestinal dysbiosis), SIBO, candida	Diet: anti-inflammatory; possible gluten, dairy or corn free. Supplements: glutamine, probiotics (VSL #3), curcumin, omega 3
Excess pitta, stomach–small intestine meridian imbalance, spleen qi deficiency	Diet: low FODMAPs, GAPS, modified candida diet. Supplements: probiotics, berberine, 5-HTP

Chart 2

Symptom	Definition	Possible Gut Causes
Alopecia areata	Autoimmune reaction causing localized, discreet hair loss	Food allergies and intolerances, candida
Dermatitis herpetiformis	Rash often found with celiac disease	Gluten intolerance, SIBO
Chronic fatigue immune deficiency syndrome	Persistent fatigue lasting for six months or more that is not relieved by rest	Leaky gut, SIBO, candida, food allergies and intolerances, low SigA
Erythema nodosum	Tender, painful lumps on the front of the legs, often reddish in color	Leaky gut, SIBO, candida, food allergies and intolerances, low SigA. Often secondary to inflammatory changes in the gut.
Fibromyalgia	Chronic, widespread pain and tenderness in muscles and joints	Food allergies, intolerances, leaky gut
Pyoderma gangrenosum	Ulcerations on the skin, often secondary to autoimmune illnesses	Malabsorption
Restless leg syndrome	An urge to move the legs that is often uncontrollable; typically occurs at night, disturbing sleep	Nutritional deficiencies secondary to leaky gut, malabsorption
Rosacea	Inflammatory skin condition often associated with redness, flushing and pustules or papules	Food allergies and intolerances, candida
Vitiligo	Autoimmune skin reaction resulting in skin depigmentation	Food allergies, intolerances, SIBO, malabsorption, low levels of stomach acid (achlorhydria)

Conventional Treatment	Integrative Medicine Diagnosis	Integrative Treatment
Localized steroid injections	Liver/kidney disharmony, heart/bladder disharmony, spleen deficiency, nutritional deficiency, Indralupta	Thyroid evaluation, nutritional evaluation and supplements, GI evaluation for candida and SIBO, gut dysfunction, food allergies, intolerances
Gluten avoidance	Excess pitta, spleen meridian disharmony, damp heat	Gluten avoidance, rebuild gut microbiology
Antidepressants, medications to relieve anxiety and/or to promote sleep, anti-viral medications	Deficiency: yin, yang, blood, qi, vata	Correct the spleen deficiency through diet, warming herbs, correct leaky gut, food allergies, intolerances
NSAIDs	Associated disease: inflammation, excess heat, spleen deficiency	Fix diet: food allergies, intolerances, dispel heat through herbs, acupuncture
Pain medications, antidepressants	Kidney qi deficiency, spleen liver imbalance, damp heat, blood stasis, excess vata	Liver detoxification, nutritional support, anti-inflammatory diet, food allergies, intolerances, hormone support
Wound care, dressing changes, steroids, topical immunosuppressants (tacrolimus)	Inflammation, excess heat, spleen deficiency	Wound care, decrease inflammation through anti-inflammatory diet, supplements, treat infection
Avoidance of alcohol, caffeine, nicotine, use of medications like dopamine agonists and benzodiazepines	Excess vata, kidney qi deficiency	Nutritional support, correct deficiencies, malabsorption
Steroids, antibiotics, immunosuppressants	Excess pitta, excess qi, liver stomach excess	Dietary evaluation, gut-based illness, avoid specific triggers: dairy, candida most common, balance gut microbiology
UV light and medications that increase sensitivity to Ultraviolet A	Liver disharmony, excess kapha, kidney disharmony	Diet evaluation for liver detoxification, strengthening qi through nutrition herbs, clean the gut through detoxification

The Supporting Cast

DON'T DO YOUR LIVER DIRTY

The liver is critical to gut health—it's the organ in charge of helping your body eliminate ama. A clean liver functions well, breaking down fats as well as filtering harmful bacteria, toxic byproducts of hormone production, dietary irritants, and environmental chemicals from your blood.

A dirty liver? That's a different story. Imbalances in the liver meridian, which runs from the foot through the breast, account for almost 85 percent of the medical issues in my patients, from infertility to cancer.

Toxins dumped in a river don't just foul the river itself. Eventually, they reach the sea. Similarly, toxins "dumped" into the gut don't just threaten the gut. If they leak through the intestinal lining, they end up in the body and eventually the liver. That's one of the reasons why a strong gut lining is so important—it supports the liver in its crucial work of detoxification.

A dirty liver is a root cause of an unhealthy gut. In Chinese medicine, a pattern of liver deficiency is tied to spleen or digestive deficiencies. These deficiencies create hormone imbalances that can lead to irregular menstrual cycles, infertility, and menopausal symptoms such as hot flashes and night sweats. A liver overwhelmed by toxins can also raise the risk of Alzheimer's disease, Parkinson's disease, and multiple sclerosis.

A dirty liver is a root cause of other diseases as well. (Remember, in Chinese medicine, the liver meridian runs right through the breast, and breast cancer is thought to originate in the liver.) The liver's toxic load may even contribute to the epidemic of obesity that's overtaken the Western world. Research suggests that the chemicals in our food and the chemicals in our environment may contribute to obesity by damaging the liver's ability to eliminate such toxins.

Dirty livers also tend to be clogged by fat that the body is unable to metabolize. Fatty liver disease, or nonalcoholic steatohepatitis (NASH), occurs when fat builds up in the liver. You may experience abdominal pain, but more often you won't know the damage your liver has sustained—untreated, fatty liver disease can lead to cirrhosis (scar tissue) or liver failure. People who are overweight or obese and/or diabetic often develop fatty livers. While the disease usually develops in middle age, it now increasingly affects children.

I see more and more fatty livers in my overweight patients. When they come in with pain in the right upper side of their abdomens, I send them for a CT or an ultrasound. In scans, a fatty liver shows up as white as snow. The white is an overload of too much dietary fat. The fat literally covers their livers, because there was nowhere else for it to go. The rest of the digestive system couldn't handle the amount, so it ended up in the liver.

The only treatment for fatty liver disease? Clean living. Typically, I prescribe a liver cleanup plan, which includes one of my Green Juice Blends (see pages 81–83). I may also put patients with fatty livers on a more structured liver detox plan. That 7- to 10-day plan features a "clean" diet and herbs and supplements that support liver detoxification, such as milk thistle and dandelion greens. Days 1–3 of the 21-Day Belly Fix plan feature such a liver cleanup component.

I once treated a woman who had previously been diagnosed with a fatty liver, caused by years of taking medications to treat her depression and high cholesterol. She came to me because her original doctor had told her that the damage to her liver was permanent. After just three months of a liver-cleansing diet, exercise, and specific liver-detoxifying herbs and supplements, I sent her for a repeat CT scan. The fat surrounding her liver was gone.

THE GALLBLADDER AND PANCREAS: GOING STEADY

In conventional medicine, it's nothing to pluck out a gallbladder, and the pancreas and liver aren't even considered digestive organs. But in ancient healing traditions, these guys are crucial digestive-system players.

The tiny, pear-shaped gallbladder beneath your liver is the holding tank for a greenish-yellow fluid called bile. During digestion, the gallbladder releases bile, made by the liver, into ducts that lead to the small intestine. There, bile breaks down, or emulsifies, the large globules of fats in chyme into smaller globs that are easier for the small intestine to digest. In Chinese medicine, the gallbladder meridian travels up the side of the leg, runs through the gallbladder, and wraps around the ear, forehead, and scalp. A gallbladder issue can cause problems anywhere along that path, from gall-stones and hormone imbalances to high cholesterol and migraines.

Nestled between the stomach and the spine and partially behind the stomach, the pancreas is six inches long and shaped like a tadpole. (It even has a "head" and a "tail"!) The enzymes this organ makes help metabolize food and maintain a proper gut pH, which helps prevent ama. The hormones it produces, such as insulin, work together to maintain the proper level of sugar in the blood. Your body uses that sugar, called glucose, for energy.

Insulin helps cells absorb and use glucose. But excess weight, a sedentary lifestyle, and other unhealthy lifestyle practices can exhaust the pancreas, which reduces the body's ability to use insulin effectively. The result: *insulin resistance*. That's when glucose builds up in the blood instead of being absorbed by the cells as it should. Insulin resistance can lead to pre-diabetes or type 2 diabetes, which significantly increases the risk of a heart attack or stroke. It's worth noting that these diseases of inflammation are triggered by dramatic changes in insulin regulation.

and diseases that research suggests have digestive causes. (Many of these include diseases of the skin as well as several other diseases that often leave conventional doctors mystified.)

If you have any of the symptoms in either chart, please schedule an appointment with your doctor, and bring this book with you. If they downplay either your symptoms or the information in these charts, search for a physician who specializes in integrative medicine. There is help available! You just have to find it.

three

The Brain in Your Belly

Some of my favorite patients are those who visited my practice the first few days it was open. Their trust in me and willingness to learn with me stay with me to this day. Michael, in his early twenties, was one of these patients.

Born in Atlanta but a Boston transplant, Michael flew to Atlanta seeking treatment for Crohn's disease, with which he was diagnosed the year before. (A friend of his from Atlanta had referred him to me.)

As a management consultant, Michael lived an insanely imbalanced lifestyle, working twelve-hour days and most weekends, with lots of travel. Many young people find a fast-paced life filled with travel exhilarating. Not Michael. The stress and brutal hours of his job turned him into a pale, thin bundle of nerves. If he ate, it was takeout—no time to cook fresh, whole food or even to order it. Sleeping just three or four hours a night didn't help, either.

Eventually, this physically and emotionally punishing lifestyle took its toll. A year into his job, Michael developed diarrhea and noticed blood in his stools. He waited three months (!) before seeing a doctor, as his symptoms grew steadily worse. Ultimately, a gastroenterologist diagnosed Crohn's disease.

I gave him a thorough workup. No food allergies, but there it was—a leaky gut, along with a Vitamin D deficiency. Further, blood tests showed that his morning levels of the stress hormone cortisol were high, suggesting adrenal fatigue. What this young man needed was rest—and a 21-Day Belly Fix to heal his leaky gut.

For the next three months, Michael flew into Atlanta for acupuncture treatment. Back in Boston, he swapped those overloaded work schedule for yoga classes and full nights of sleep.

By his third round of acupuncture, Michael was feeling much better—fewer bouts of diarrhea and abdominal pain and very little blood in his stools. At this point, he realized he had a decision to make: his high-flying career or his health. He quit his job, moved home to Atlanta, found a less stressful (but still interesting) job, and continued his acupuncture treatments and yoga. Today, he's a new man—healthy, relaxed, and full of life. And as long as he manages his stress, he'll remain that way.

I tell that story because while the eyes may be the windows of your soul, your gut—more specifically, the brain in your gut—holds the wisdom of your body. Formally known as the enteric nervous system (ENS), your gut-brain can run your digestive system without any help from your head-brain, yet your two brains "chatter" constantly. Those intuitive "gut feelings" begin in the belly-brain, too, the result of electrical signals generated by nerve cells in its lining.

Part of the nervous system that evolved more than five hundred million years ago, the gut-brain rivals the head-brain in its sophistication and complexity. Scientists have just begun to fathom the relationship between the two.

What we do know: There's a link between the belly-brain and the central nervous system—called the gut-brain axis—that coordinates the brain, intestinal tract, and the hormone and immune systems that maintain gut function. What this means is that a mind in distress signals the gut, and a gut in distress tells the brain; your intestinal distress can be the cause of anxiety, stress, or depression—or a reaction to it.

Chinese and Ayurvedic medicine show an awareness, if not a scientific understanding, of the gut-brain. (For example, an anxious person needs to "cool" the mind by warming and nourishing the gut.) The intuitive wisdom in these ancient systems echoes the most cutting-edge research. Some researchers are investigating how the second brain mediates the body's immune response. (Remember, 70 percent of our immune system resides in the gut.) Others study how the gut microbiota "communicates" with cells in the ENS.

Yet others are focused on the role of brain chemicals called neurotransmitters. Each neurotransmitter plays specific roles in regulating mood, appetite, and memory. Think of neurotransmitters as the chemical "words" that nerve cells use to "talk" to each other and to the cells they control.

In a healthy gut-brain, neurotransmitters are in balance, helping your mind and body function at their peak. If, however, these crucial chemicals are knocked off-kilter, as they frequently are by genetic, digestive, and lifestyle factors, symptoms develop and then progress to illness. Even more astounding, the ways that your brain and body may react to a neurotransmitter imbalance may differ from mine. For instance, a deficiency in serotonin (see page 46) may cause depression in one person, panic attacks in another, and uncontrollable food cravings in someone else.

The patients who come to see me with what they consider to be a mental illness are always shocked when I begin their treatment with a 21-Day Belly Fix. That's because neurotransmitter balance requires the right mix of gut function, nutrients, and hormone balance. This chapter examines five conditions most commonly linked to an imbalance of neurotransmitters in the belly-brain: weight gain, stress, anxiety/depression, focus/attention, and IBS. We'll examine each in detail. But first, it's vital to understand how the gut-brain works as well as the neurotransmitters that play such a critical role in its functioning.

Your Second Brain and Its Chemical Helpers

As you'll recall from chapter 2, the first two branches of your autonomic nervous system—which controls body processes we virtually never think about, including heart rate, blood pressure, breathing, and digestion—are

Science, Meet Wisdom

Thousands of years ago, the practitioners of Chinese and Ayurvedic medicine didn't know that the gut-brain existed. But they wisely identified the digestive system as the key to well-being, and their healing practices reflected it.

In both systems, imbalances in the body's energy systems (in Ayurveda the chakras, in Chinese medicine the meridians) can cause digestive issues, which are often traced to worry and stress. Two different systems, one unifying principle. Interesting, no? But it gets even more interesting.

As I've mentioned previously, in Chinese medicine, the spleen meridian rules digestion. A pregnant woman consumed by stress is in danger of depleting her spleen or digestive qi and may bear a child with digestive issues. Yes, it sounds pretty out there. Except that it happened to me.

In 2008, I was pregnant with my son Kubby and had given birth to my daughter, Rania, just six months before. It was a no-good, very bad time. I was working in the ER, caring for an infant, and starting my integrative practice, all while Vik was starting his practice.

I wish I could say that the stress of that time is but a distant memory. But even years later, the memories are fresh. But true to my pitta-dominant nature, I powered through and gave birth to my beautiful son.

Kubby was perfect in every way, except for one thing: From the day he was born, he suffered from severe reflux. Every feeding came back up. This pattern continued for months. As a toddler, he lay on his belly, unable to eat past a certain point. When he was three, I tested him for food allergies and intolerances and leaky gut. My tests showed that, like mine, his gut cannot tolerate gluten.

Immediately I put him on a gluten-free diet and a digestive regimen of glutamine and probiotics. He is doing better. From below the 3rd percentile for his height and weight at age two, he is now in the 10th percentile. As he continues to heal, the hope is that he will make it into the 25th percentile.

While I understand that my son has a medical condition, I am haunted by the thought that my extreme stress while I was carrying him may have been a factor. Could it be that I depleted my own spleen qi, which created weak spleen qi in my child? I believe it's possible. So you see, the power and influence of the gut, recognized thousands of years ago by completely different systems of medicine, play out over and over again today. Feel free to raise your eyebrow at traditional systems of medicine, but do me a favor— take good care of your gut.

fight-or-flight and rest-and-digest. The third branch is the ENS— basically a bundle of neurons embedded in the walls of your gut. These nerve cells are the basic building blocks of the brain and nervous system.

But that simple description of the belly-brain belies its complexity. It comes equipped with a network of one hundred million neurons, more than are in your spine. To do its work, it uses more than thirty neurotransmitters, the same ones the brain uses. One of these is serotonin, which helps regulate mood, sleep, and digestion, among other processes. Serotonin is often called "the feel-good hormone." As you'll see, it's much more than that.

The gut-brain monitors digestion, detects nutrients, and regulates the functions of the GI tract. Neurotransmitters—those chemical "words" in the language of neurons—play a vital part in all of these roles as well as in the two-way communication between gut-brain and head-brain. To get their chemical messages from one neuron to another, neurotransmitters "leap" across tiny gaps between neurons called synapses.

Thanks in large part to neurotransmitters, your gut-brain is in constant communication with your head-brain. The "dialogue" between gut and brain takes place through the vagus nerve, *vagus* being the Latin word for "wandering." True to its name, the vagus nerve starts in your brain stem, meanders through organs in your neck and chest, and ends in your belly. It's the vagus nerve that keeps the gut and brain "connected." Think of this long nerve as a Facebook page where the gut and the brain constantly post "status updates." When things are running well, the messages can be thought of as a quick update. However, if the gut is unhappy, it lets the brain know. A constant onslaught of negative messages from the gut can eventually affect the neuron activity in the brain and lead to anxiety, depression, and sleep disturbances. In short: When your brain chemistry is off, your gut can suffer, too. And when your gut's out of balance, your mind, mood, and health can be affected.

Now that you know what the gut-brain is, let's turn to the conditions that can result from unbalanced brain chemicals. These include weight gain, stress, anxiety and depression, focus and attention, and irritable bowel syndrome (IBS). Too much or too little of any one neurotransmitter can be the domino that gets the whole stack tumbling, affecting critical body functions. Let's see how:

STRESS

When Hormones Collide

We've all experienced the familiar signs of stress—sweaty palms, racing heart, momentary shortness of breath. What's fascinating is that, despite these common symptoms, stress "expresses itself" in ways that are unique to us, and often we know intuitively when we are out of balance.

If you associate stress with disharmony, you're thinking like a practitioner of Chinese or Ayurvedic medicine. Indeed, in both traditional medicine systems, stress triggers imbalances. In Chinese medicine, stress knocks the heart and liver meridians—those energy pathways mentioned in chapter 1—out of harmony. In Ayurvedic medicine, stress causes pitta energy to overpower the other doshas, increasing digestive heat. This heat weakens agni, creates ama, and attacks the gut.

But what traditional healers didn't know—and what you may be unaware of—is that your hormones, which work in concert to regulate your mind and mood, reflect this disharmony. Stress produced by the demands of job and family; physical stresses like dieting and lack of sleep; distress triggered by worries about money or health—every day, stressors like these induce our adrenal glands to produce stress hormones such as adrenaline and cortisol. These stress hormones play a key role in the fight-or-flight response.

Normally, we require only small blasts of stress-hormone "fuel" to awaken us in the morning and keep us alert and focused throughout the day.

But if our stress never wanes—if our bodies are continually in the grips of the fight-or-flight response—the adrenals are forced to pump out high amounts of these stress hormones constantly. Eventually, under this much stress, the adrenals can no longer function properly. Basically, they burn out. The resulting adrenal fatigue affects not only our short-term response to stress, but our adrenal glands' ability to balance other hormones that affect our health and well-being, such as cortisol, thyroid hormone, and insulin.

Because we each perceive "threats" differently, and each of us responds to stress in a unique way, I see adrenal fatigue in executives and stay-at-home moms alike. In all cases, their adrenal glands have simply burned out, and they exhibit a wide variety of symptoms, from food cravings or a foggy brain to a literal inability to get out of bed in the morning. Adrenal imbalance can be a contributing factor in other, seemingly unrelated health issues, including depression, chronic allergies, and infertility.

Many of my patients who suffer from adrenal fatigue also are plagued by powerful food cravings and weight gain. A stressed brain seeks instant gratification to feel better. Food can be that quick fix. Under chronic stress, the gut releases ghrelin, frequently dubbed "the hunger hormone." Along with amping up appetite, ghrelin increases dopamine levels. As you might imagine, you want to stay on the right side of a hormone that triggers appetite, is unleashed by stress, and helps release dopamine.

The hormones associated with stress can affect digestion, too. For example, an excess of adrenaline can cause gas and flatulence, which aren't funny when you're stressed. Diarrhea may be an issue as well. Or you may be one of the rare people who, under stress, develops constipation—the result of a slowdown in gut motility. (To add insult to injury, you get the gas, too.)

Whether you need to go more often or less often, your health can suffer. Diarrhea or constipation can lead to malabsorption or leaky gut. In turn, leaky gut can cause inflammation and nutritional deficiencies and

The Serotonin Connection

You may have read that serotonin promotes restful sleep and a mellow, even-keel mood, and that's true. But a lot of people also think that a chemical that so influences mind and mood must be made in the brain.

Surprise—a whopping 95 percent of the serotonin in your body is manufactured in your gut, with assistance from special cells embedded in the intestinal wall. These enterochromaffin cells produce the precursor to serotonin: the amino acid 5-hydroxytryptophan, or 5-HTP. It's 5-HTP that determines whether serotonin is broken down and used or built up but ignored.

Nor does serotonin affect only mood and sleep. This neurotransmitter plays a critical role in digestion. Digestion begins when enterochromaffin cells secrete serotonin into the intestinal walls. Serotonin receptors signal neurons to start the flow of digestive enzymes. Serotonin also affects motility, or how fast food moves through your gut, as well as the sensitivity of your belly to sensations like fullness or pain.

Serotonin balance is determined by genetics and gut health. Stress, medications, or poor diet may unbalance the gut, which means that it may make either too much serotonin or too little. Research has connected excess serotonin in the gut to depression, inattention, and even autism and too little serotonin to anxiety, blood sugar imbalances, and hormone imbalances. What's more, research now suggests that serotonin levels are a significant factor in IBS (see page 50).

The bottom line: if the gut makes enough serotonin and that serotonin is metabolized effectively, stress and food cravings can be managed without too much of a problem. If it doesn't, depression, comfort-food cravings, and weight gain may be the result. The serotonin connection is more proof that an out-of-whack gut affects not just our bellies but our entire state of being as well.

Pharmaceutical companies have created a vast array of serotonin-modulating medications meant to treat depression, anxiety, IBS, and attention-deficit disorder/attention-deficit hyperactivity disorder (ADD/ADHD). I prescribe them sparingly, knowing that the 21-Day Belly Fix and a few supplements can improve, if not resolve, issues with serotonin metabolism.

lead to imbalances in important hormones, including thyroid hormone, estrogen, and progesterone.

After such troubling news, I am happy to tell you that you may not need antidepressants or anti-anxiety medications to get a handle on stress. Conquering its negative effects on your life can be as simple as giving your gut what it needs to manage stress and therefore minimize its impact on your life and your mood.

ANXIETY/DEPRESSION

Gut-Level Emotions

Nearly 18 percent of Americans experience mild or major depression, another 18 percent anxiety disorders. Both involve a combination of genetic, biological, environmental, and psychological factors. However, there's amazing research that supports the link between digestive health and depression and anxiety. (ADD/ADHD and autism spectrum disorders, too—I'll get to that below.)

The upshot? When patients come to me about anxiety or depression, I don't give them a prescription for an antidepressant or anti-anxiety medication. I give them a 21-Day Belly Fix. Remember the gut-brain axis: Treating gut dysfunction can improve mood by altering brain chemistry, and managing anxiety and depression can improve gut issues.

When it comes to depression and anxiety, a variety of gut factors may be at play. An imbalanced gut microbiota, for one. Numerous studies have found that psychological stress suppresses "good" gut bacteria, increasing susceptibility to infection and causing gut inflammation. Further, substances produced by the gut during infection, called inflammatory cytokines, disrupt brain neurochemistry, thereby increasing susceptibility to anxiety and depression. This may be why so many with Crohn's disease, IBS, and other chronic GI disorders suffer from anxiety and depression.

Leaky gut, which can lead to nutritional deficiencies and neurotransmitter imbalances, may contribute to depression and anxiety, too. As dopamine and serotonin are imbalanced, anxiety and depression ensue. A

2008 study published in *Neuroendocrinology Letters* found that—compared to non-depressed volunteers—the immune systems of people with major depression were more likely to mount a response to gut bacteria that had "invaded" the bloodstream. Activation of the inflammatory response system plays a role in the pathology of depression, the study found.

What about anxiety? Well, the chronic, low-grade inflammation caused by a leaky gut stresses the body. In response to this stress, the body is flooded with the stress hormone cortisol. One consequence of a body stuck in fight-or-flight mode? Anxiety. Other studies suggest a link between allergy or intolerance to food additives (such as monosodium glutamate or MSG), artificial sweeteners (such as aspartame), and colorings or preservatives (such as tartrazine, benzoates, and sorbates).

FOCUS AND ATTENTION

Ancient Medicine Means Fewer "Meds"

When they first come to see me, many of my patients—both adults and children—are taking medication for ADD/ADHD. Adults tell me that these medications make them feel "better" and help them get more done. Parents tell me that these medications directly impact their children's grades and school performance.

There is an ongoing debate among researchers and physicians about whether ADD/ADHD is a disease of modern civilization or just went unrecognized in the past. However, a growing number of researchers are beginning to see these conditions—along with sensory processing disorders like pervasive developmental disorders (PDD), autism, Asperger syndrome, and obsessive-compulsive disorder (OCD)—as inflammatory bowel diseases rather than pure neurological challenges.

This doesn't surprise me. Neurotransmitter balance is dictated by gut balance. Our steady diet of processed, genetically modified "food" has unbalanced our gut flora and poked holes in our gut linings. Our dependence on antibiotics and overreliance on vaccinations in childhood have created the "hygiene hypothesis"—the possibility that we have changed our gut flora more in the last fifty years than at any other time in history. All of these factors alter neurotransmitter balance. The rates of ADD/ADHD and autism are rising, and it's my belief that gut factors are at play.

I've treated thousands of adults and children diagnosed with ADD/ADHD. What I've learned is that four neurotransmitters are associated with ADD/ADHD: dopamine, serotonin, gamma-aminobutyric acid (GABA), and norepinephrine. All of them are made in the gut and all of them are essential to the ENS. Too much dopamine or norepinephrine is likely to cause hyperactivity. Too little serotonin or GABA, and inattentiveness tends to be the issue. And low levels of dopamine tend to result in a constant state of brain fog. Rebalancing these neurotransmitters is essential.

I apply the principles of Chinese medicine and its "Five Elements" concept in working with patients with attention problems. For example, a child or adult who is a wood type typically exhibits more aggression and is often deficient in dopamine. I do prescribe low-dose ADD medications for this type. On the other hand, fire types often are deficient in serotonin, are typically very sensitive, and do poorly on stimulant medications.

First, I "type" each patient as one of the five elements. Then I use blood and urine neurotransmitter testing to confirm my Chinese medicine diagnosis. Finally, I customize their treatment to their type. Once I find the neurotransmitter or neurotransmitters that are out of balance, my patients and I team up to design a treatment plan. Frequently, such plans include a customized diet to rebalance those neurotransmitters and repair the gut lining so that it will absorb brain-friendly B vitamins as well as amino acids crucial to brain function, such as tryptophan and taurine. Fermented foods can help rebalance their gut flora with probiotics and therefore help resolve symptoms such as brain fog, inattention, and disorganization. (We'll discuss probiotics in chapter 4.) My goal is to show my patients how to embrace and balance their type with diet, supplements, breathing, and other mind-body techniques.

It may sound too good to be true, but the 21-Day Belly Fix can begin your journey to healing from ADD/ADHD. Diet really makes a difference. Time after time, simple dietary changes—eliminating gluten (see page 51) or dairy, limiting sugar—produce sudden and often dramatic improvements in my patients' focus and attention. If they have gastrointestinal symptoms, those improve, too.

IBS

Different Symptoms, Different Serotonin Levels

In no other disease is the role of the gut-brain as blatant as in IBS, which is characterized by abdominal pain and changes in bowel habits—you eliminate either too much or too little. This condition used to be called terrible names, including "nervous colon" or "spastic bowel." Thankfully, the name was changed—doctors and researchers now know that IBS is not "all in your head."

First, the facts: IBS is known as a "functional" GI disorder, meaning that its symptoms are caused by changes in how the GI tract works. The pain or discomfort typically occurs with a change in stool frequency or consistency, and people usually feel better after they "go." Doctors typically diagnose IBS when abdominal pain or discomfort occurs at least three times a month for three months and all other potential causes have been ruled out. While IBS symptoms can be considerable, they don't damage the bowel as much as inflammatory bowel diseases such as Crohn's disease or ulcerative colitis do.

No single cause of IBS has been identified. Contributing factors include small intestine bacterial overgrowth (SIBO), food intolerances, and stress. However, more and more gastroenterologists are identifying a change in brain-gut communication or serotonin as a factor. A substance called 5-hydroxytryptophan, or 5-HTP, is the building block for serotonin. It's thought that too many 5-HTP receptors in the gut lead to diarrhea; too few, to constipation. Diet, stress, and microbiology in the belly determine whether serotonin will be released by these gut cells, broken down, or ignored.

For example, people with IBS with constipation as their major symptom often have lower-than-normal levels of serotonin. The muscles in their rectums are less reactive to serotonin, causing stools that are hard or

Are You Getting "Glutened"?

Your fingers go numb. Your get a killer headache or an itchy rash. You become edgy or moody, you're suddenly hell on wheels—or you can't put two thoughts together.

There's a good chance you've been "glutened"—and you may not even realize it.

Strange but true—a simple protein in wheat, rye, and barley can trigger the misery of celiac disease (CD) and gluten sensitivity. (To distinguish it from the full-blown disease, its formal name is "non-celiac gluten sensitivity.") It's estimated that 18 million Americans are gluten-sensitive—six times the number with CD.

The difference between CD and gluten sensitivity is the response of the immune system. The immune systems of people with gluten sensitivity view gluten as an invader and "attack" gluten with inflammation. In CD, gluten triggers the immune system to attack the body's own tissue—in this case, the intestinal lining.

The only way to know if you have gluten sensitivity is to test negatively for CD or wheat allergy—typically an expensive and drawn-out proposition. So if I suspect gluten sensitivity in my patients, I simply have them stop eating foods containing gluten for a time. If their symptoms improve, gluten sensitivity is a reasonable assumption.

As I have mentioned, I am gluten sensitive. In hindsight, that explained a lot. While gluten sensitivity doesn't cause the small intestine damage CD does, its symptoms are similar—abdominal pain, bloating, diarrhea, constipation, headaches, joint pain, and chronic fatigue. But gluten sensitivity also messes with your mind and mood, causing "foggy mind," issues with focus and attention, irritability, and depression.

Most mainstream doctors aren't familiar with the gluten/mood connection. However, research links major depression, along with chronic, mild depression, to gluten sensitivity and CD, so depression can be a red flag for undiagnosed CD. A 2012 study conducted on women with CD, published in the medical journal *Chronic Illness*, found that 37 percent suffered from clinical depression. In another study of children with CD, researchers in Italy found that rates of depression ranged from almost 9 percent in boys to 14 percent in girls.

Though I've followed a gluten-free diet for years, at times I trip up and get "glutened"—that is, accidentally eat a food containing gluten. The consequences of even the tiniest crumb of the stuff sneaking into my diet are hell. My high-energy self disappears, replaced by a "shadow self" who is depressed and lethargic and suffers from an embarrassing number of "brain farts."

My son, Kubby, is also gluten-sensitive—his digestive-based symptoms started at birth, and I tested him when he was three. But ingesting gluten affects his disposition as well. While he did not demonstrate clear symptoms of anxiety or depression, as some people might, when he gets "glutened" he is a holy terror—irritable and difficult to manage. Believe me, I've dealt with my fair share of temper tantrums!

lumpy. Others with IBS, who have diarrhea as their primary symptom, have been shown to have serotonin levels that are higher than normal. Their rectums are more reactive, and more likely to empty too early. Significantly, people with IBS are more likely to suffer from anxiety, depression, and stress than people who don't.

Interestingly, IBS—considered a modern disease—is mentioned in both Chinese medicine and Ayurveda. In Chinese medicine, IBS is a liver-spleen meridian imbalance caused by a deficiency in qi or overall energy. As the spleen weakens, the liver meridian becomes overactive, stressing the other meridians and contributing to further imbalance. This imbalance causes a weakened digestive system or dampness, cold, and stasis. Ayurvedic texts describe IBS as grahani and define grahani as an imbalance between the pitta and vata doshas. In both systems of medicine, the main course of treatment is a diet of easily digestible foods and herbs or supplements to aid digestion.

The 21-Day Belly Fix—along with supplements, herbs, acupuncture or abdominal wall massage—improves the symptoms of most of my patients with IBS. I never prescribe medications for IBS. As an integrative doctor, my goal is to dig for the underlying cause, not mask or treat the symptoms.

four

Diet-Free Weight Loss

By now, you've learned about all the things the 21-Day Belly Fix can cure, but you may be most interested in the one we've saved for last: the flabby belly itself! Not a day goes by when a patient does not ask me how they can lose weight. The four steps below provide the answer; then the 21-Day Belly Fix, in the next chapter, puts them in action. You're just a few pages away from losing that first ten pounds, I promise. It'll melt away when you:

1. MASTER YOUR CHEMISTRY

Want to lose weight? Tell me the tale of how you became overweight to begin with. There are clues in that story. Yes, poor diet and exercise habits can be major factors. However, so can hormone imbalances and, especially, emotionally driven overeating triggered by stress—an ongoing relationship issue, career or financial worries, or other unresolved life issues. That constant stress drives poor food choices, which in turn affect the balance of key neurotransmitters involved in regulating appetite. These neurotransmitters are serotonin and dopamine.

Serotonin acts as both a mood stabilizer and an appetite suppressant.

It's been found to curb cravings, to prompt that "I'm full" feeling of satiety, and to promote a state of calm alertness.

It's long been known that carbohydrate foods, but not protein foods, increase serotonin production. The reason has to do with the amino acid tryptophan, serotonin's building block. Put simply, the tryptophan in protein foods must compete with over twenty other amino acids to cross from the bloodstream into the brain. The tryptophan in carbohydrate foods, however, has no such competition. Ignored by the hormone insulin, tryptophan stays in the bloodstream and makes it into the brain, where it's quickly converted to soothing, appetite-stomping serotonin. However, stress depletes serotonin in the brain. If you don't raise it, you may find yourself gorging on pizza and cupcakes.

What about dopamine? Think of it as the Rick James of neurotransmitters —it wants to party. Strongly associated with reward mechanisms in the brain, dopamine urges us to seek out things that make us feel good—sex, social interaction, art, or other natural pleasures that help ensure our survival. The gut-brain produces almost half of the body's supply.

Poor food choices, the wrong microbiology, stress, medications, or chronic illness can affect the gut-brain—and dopamine production. An imbalance in dopamine can disrupt our ability to feel satisfied, both in an emotional sense and in a food sense. As a result, dopamine-deficient people can go on a kind of dopamine safari, seeking bliss not in healthy pleasures but in illicit drugs (heroin or cocaine; also alcohol and nicotine) or in food. Presto—weight gain.

In a study published in the medical journal *The Lancet,* researchers scanned the brains of ten obese and ten normal-weight people. Specifically, they wanted to know if the brains of their obese volunteers showed normal dopamine activity. So the team measured the availability of a specific dopamine receptor known as D2.

Their findings? Obese people had fewer dopamine receptors. Moreover, the more obese their volunteers were, the fewer D2 receptors they had. In fact, the team noted that the brains of their obese volunteers and those of people addicted to illicit drugs both have fewer dopamine receptors than the brains of normal people.

It may be that drug use or compulsive overeating lowers the number of dopamine receptors, or it may be that some of us are born with fewer dopamine receptors. If the latter turns out to be true, the implications are stunning. Think about it. If those who compulsively seek illicit drugs or food are born with fewer dopamine receptors, they may not respond to natural pleasures that bliss out those born with adequate numbers. This just might explain the drive to consume substances that trigger dopamine release: heroin or ice cream, crack cocaine or bacon cheeseburgers.

Many of my patients who need to lose weight for health reasons do shed those extra pounds. I think there are a variety of reasons for this. First, rebalancing neurotransmitters that regulate mood and appetite means that you are less likely to use food to relieve stress and negative emotions such as depression and anxiety. The plan also helps rebalance the bacteria in your digestive system, and there's now compelling evidence that a healthy mix of gut bacteria may contribute to a healthy weight or promote weight loss.

2. BALANCE YOUR BACTERIA

What makes you you? A philosopher would respond quite differently than a biologist. But the fact is, your body contains ten times more bacteria than cells. No need to do the math. The sweet, smart, wonderful you, inside and out, is crawling with 100 trillion microbes.

Yes, it's a bit creepy. But it's exactly as nature intends.

The moment you left your mother's body, microbes colonized every square inch of you, including your gut. *Especially* your gut. The bacteria "stew" bubbling in your belly—a veritable rainforest of species, called the gut microbiota—helps digest food, synthesizes nutrients, and partners with the immune system to help protect you from invaders. This lively mass of microbes plays a role in fighting a wide-ranging list of diseases, allergies like asthma and hay fever, inflammatory conditions from IBD to heart disease and cancer, and even obesity. There's also evidence that that abundant and diverse species of bacteria in our gut influences our moods and even our personalities.

While some of these bacterial species in our gut stew can make us sick, most are "friendlies," and they are intimately entwined with our health. And our modern way of life has altered it in ways that are concerning.

For example, one species of gut bacteria has made its home in the human gut for *ten thousand years*. If you have a peptic ulcer or know someone who does, you know its name: *Helicobacter pylori*. But it's disappearing from modern colonies. You'd think that this would be a good thing. In some ways, it is—rates of ulcers and stomach cancer are on the wane. But there's a catch—*H. pylori* also appears to protect against asthma, allergies, and some cancers. Further, there's evidence that its disappearance from the human gut might increase the risk of obesity. Research shows a strong relationship between *H. pylori* and levels of the "hunger hormone" ghrelin. In a study of ninety-two people published in the journal *BMC Gastroenterology*, killing off *H. pylori* with antibiotics and other medications to treat their peptic ulcers led to significant weight gain. Killing *H. pylori* is a part of diagnosing and treating peptic ulcers.

The take-home message? Yes, it's important to destroy bacteria that make us sick. But it's equally important to nurture and nourish those that promote our health and vitality. In this chapter, you'll learn how the wrong balance of gut bacteria can affect your health and weight, and how to balance it again. The result will be a lifetime of weight control—no fad diets required.

A Delicate Balance, Often Disrupted

Like your gastrointestinal system and your belly-brain, that bacterial rainforest in your gut is extraordinarily complex. It includes at least a thousand different species of bacteria made up of more than three million genes—150 times more than those in the human genome.

Your gut flora is also extremely sensitive. Anything that upsets your body's delicate balance can upset the abundance and diversity of your gut bacteria. When that happens, you may not have enough "good guys" in your gut, and the potentially health-threatening bugs may gain the advantage.

Is Your "Gut Stew" in Balance?

Some people with microbial imbalance in the gut (gut dysbiosis) have no symptoms. However, there are typically some signs that something's amiss in the digestive system. Foul-smelling poop is one of them. While all bowel movements have odor, it shouldn't run you (or your family) out of the bathroom.

Other symptoms include:

- Bad breath
- Body odor
- Bloating and gas
- Nausea
- Constipation

The good news? The 21-Day Belly Fix can help rebalance the bacteria in your digestive system, reigniting your digestive fire and—with it—your health, energy, and vitality.

The most common reason for bacterial imbalance in the gut, called dysbiosis, is the high-sugar, high-fat Western diet. For example, research has shown that refined sugars bring out an overgrowth of bad bacteria like *Clostridium difficile,* a bacterium that can cause symptoms that range from bouts of diarrhea to life-threatening inflammation of the colon. Diet is so important to a healthy balance of gut bacteria that I discuss it at length later in the chapter. For now, let's examine other factors that can upset that balance.

STRESS. As you learned in chapter 3, chronic stress forces the adrenal glands to pump out high amounts of stress hormones such as cortisol. This constant "bath" of stress hormones wears down the immune system and disrupts the gut's bacterial balance. Psychological stress has also been found to reduce the production of mucus in the gut, which helps keep bad bacteria from sticking to the lining of the gut. Less mucus means that bad bugs find it easier to make themselves at home in your gut.

OVERUSE OF ANTIBIOTICS. Antibiotics are both life-saving drugs and indiscriminate killers. It's not the fault of antibiotics, but our overreliance on them, which has led to the looming specter of antibiotic-resistant bacteria. Along with destroying the "bad" bacteria that cause infections, antibiotics kill the gut's friendly bacteria, giving free rein to unfriendly disease-causing bacteria, viruses, yeasts, and parasites.

Recent research has shown that repeated antibiotic use wreaks havoc on the diversity and composition of the gut flora. There's also evidence that exposure to antibiotics, especially early in life, may kill off healthy bacteria that influence how we absorb nutrients into our bodies, bacteria that would otherwise keep us lean. Considering that the average child receives about a dozen courses of antibiotics, this has scary, scary implications for our children's future health.

EXCESSIVE USE OF MEDICATIONS. Prolonged use of prescription and over-the-counter medications, including antacids, acid-blockers, and antidepressants, kill both harmful and helpful bacteria in the gut, leaving it vulnerable to bacteria, parasites, viruses, and fungi. Continuous use of NSAIDs (aspirin, ibuprofen, naproxen) can also wreak havoc on your gut stew. NSAIDs work by blocking prostaglandins, chemicals that cause the inflammation associated with pain and that also trigger the body's healing process. NSAIDs block *all* prostaglandins. This means that although NSAIDs ease pain, they also block the body's healing process. Continuous use of NSAIDs blocks the digestive tract's ability to do important repair work. Eventually, the gut lining becomes inflamed and potentially leaky.

HEAVY METALS. Air, water, and soil are contaminated with heavy metals such as lead, cadmium, arsenic, chromium, and mercury. Research has linked exposure to these metals with chronic inflammation and cancer as well as significant changes in the bacterial composition of the gut. Without the right balance of bugs, heavy metals build up in the gut, and even the small amounts in the environment can be toxic. It's a vicious cycle—the more heavy metals accumulate in the gut, the more damage to its lining they cause and the more that the bacterial microbiology is altered.

The Gut Bug/Health Connection

Study after study suggests that the influence of those wriggling bugs in our guts have a far-reaching impact on our health. Here's a sampling of the discoveries.

- Mice fed the *Lactobacillus rhamnosus* bacterium—used to make foods like sourdough bread, yogurt, and cheese—showed fewer symptoms of anxiety and depression, a 2011 study published in *Proceedings of the National Academy of Science* found. This study may have implications for people—in my patients, it's clear that when fermented foods or foods high in probiotics are added to the diet, food sensitivities improve. It may be that *L. rhamnosus* heightens activity in one of the receptors for a neurotransmitter called GABA (see chapter 3), which helps regulate emotional behavior.

- Infants who lack a diverse gut flora develop more allergies by the time they hit first grade, suggests a study published in the medical journal *Pediatrics*. In this study, Danish researchers reviewed the medical records and tested stool samples of 411 infants every six months until they reached the age of six. Those who didn't have diverse colonies of gut bacteria were more likely to develop allergies, the team found. Interestingly, they were not more prone to developing asthma.

- In a 2013 review published in *Annals of Hepatology*, researchers from Italy noted that between 20 and 75 percent of patients with chronic fatty liver disease—which I discussed in chapter 2—also had an overgrowth of gut bacteria. The study also noted that probiotics may one day constitute a "new, safe, well tolerated and natural treatment" for this disease. (I'm already using them!)

- Researchers have long known that breastfeeding moms transfer the protective effects of their gut bugs to their babies. A recent study in *Environmental Microbiology* shows that important "good" bacteria arrive in babies' digestive systems from their mother's gut via breast milk.

The Weight/Bug Connection

You've heard the saying "You can never be too rich or too thin"? It makes sense, if "richness" refers to a wide diversity of bacterial species in the gut. In fact, recent research associates bacterial "richness" to better metabolic health and a healthier weight. A *low* diversity of gut bugs—bacterial "poverty," if you will—seems to raise the risk of obesity and the diseases associated with it, including type 2 diabetes.

In a study published in the journal *Nature,* an international team of researchers studied 292 Danish people's gut bacteria. Specifically, it analyzed the *gene composition* of their gut bacteria. (Even bacteria have genes!) The guts of about a quarter of the volunteers showed "bacterial poverty." Put simply, their guts showed less gene and species richness. Compared to those with bacterial richness, they carried more body fat and had higher triglycerides, cholesterol levels, and levels of insulin resistance. They also had more systemic inflammation, a characteristic of virtually all chronic diseases.

What's more, obese people with gut-bacteria "poverty" gained more body weight over time than lean volunteers, the team found. They either lacked, or had a very low population of, eight specific species of bacteria, which may have played a protective role against weight gain.

So how can you shed the pounds? Diet can help turn poverty to richness. In another study published in the same issue of *Nature,* researchers put forty-nine overweight volunteers on a calorie-restricted diet for six weeks. At the end of that time, they were placed on a different diet to maintain their weight. The researchers then studied the changes in their gut bacteria.

Strikingly, those with bacterial "poverty" at the start of the study saw their diversity increase and their metabolic markers improve. (Those already "rich" saw less improvement.) Further, eating more high-fiber fruit and vegetables increased bacterial richness and improved some clinical symptoms associated with obesity, the study found.

Taken together, the findings of both studies are clear: Low bacterial richness may adversely affect weight and metabolic health, but dietary changes may make your gut bacteria "richer" and lower the risk of chronic disease.

It's vital to understand, however, that low bacterial diversity doesn't necessarily lead to obesity. Of the 292 people in the first study, 57 percent were obese, but only 23 percent of the entire group had low genetic diversity. That means that some obese people had high bacterial diversity. (This was true in the second study as well.) Still, it seems safe to say that the "richer" people's gut flora, the healthier and slimmer they tend to be—and diet can play a significant role.

3. EAT CLEAN

Keep It Real—and Green

There's a doughnut store chain that claims that America runs on its products. Really? A high-fat, high-sugar diet can shift the balance of bacteria in the gut—for better or worse—in *one day*. How far can you run on that?

A steady diet of what I call *FINO*—"Food in Name Only"—processed food promotes the development of bacteria called firmicutes that are more effective at breaking down foods that normally pass through the body at least partially undigested. That means that you extract more calories from the foods you eat, making it easier for you to gain weight.

So let me rephrase that slogan. The *gut* runs on food. Actual food. Grown in soil (which is also full of gut-friendly bacteria). Rich in fiber, gut bacteria's favorite dish. You need only follow the simple guidelines below to keep your gut bacteria in healthy, harmonious balance. Keep them in mind as you begin the 21-Day Belly Fix in the next chapter.

Fruits and Veggies: Keep It Clean

To improve the diversity and health of your gut bugs, it's not enough to eat *more* fruits and veggies. It's vital to eat *a wide variety* of them, so that your gut benefits from their diverse types and amounts of fiber.

If you're a corn-spuds-and-peas type of person, the 21-Day Belly Fix

Obesity on Your Breath?

Your breath may betray bacterial "poverty" in your gut.

In a study published in the *Journal of Clinical Endocrinology and Metabolism,* researchers analyzed the breath of 792 people for the gases methane and hydrogen. Their volunteers fell into four categories: normal breath content, higher concentrations of methane, higher levels of hydrogen, or higher levels of both. Those with high concentrations of both gases had significantly higher BMIs and carried more body fat.

The theory is that *Methanobrevibacter smithii* feeds on the hydrogen produced by other gut bacteria. Lower hydrogen levels raise fermentation in the gut, allowing the body to absorb more nutrients—and calories—from food. So *M. smithii* may have been useful to cavemen, who ate more roughage and needed all the help they could get to extract every last calorie from their meager meals. But our diets, which are low in fiber, may have turned this asset into a liability.

will be a big change. But give it a chance. As you venture into the delicious diversity of a plant-based diet, you'll do your digestive tract a world of good. Friendly gut bugs like all types of fiber. The tougher the fiber, the harder it is to digest. From your gut stew's point of view, this is a good thing.

So eat the fibrous broccoli stalks as well as the softer crowns, the woody stalks of asparagus along with the tender tips. These harder-to-digest parts act as a kind of whisk broom to sweep your digestive tract clean. Also, when you eat veggies raw, or cook them until they're tender-crisp, your gut has to work harder to break them down. That's good "exercise" for your colon.

As you increase the variety of the plant foods you eat, be sure to include onions, garlic, asparagus, and leeks. These foods are chock-full of *prebiotics*—special types of fiber that resist digestion in the small intestine and, once they hit the colon, are fermented by our gut stew. These fibers selectively stimulate the growth and/or activity of good gut bugs.

While you're keeping your diet green, keep it real, too—with foods naturally rich in beneficial bacteria known as *probiotics*. The "friendlies" in fermented foods and beverages such as yogurt and kefir, sauerkraut, kimchi, and kombucha help replenish good gut bugs and make your gut a hostile environment for bad ones. I'll discuss probiotics—which are a natural part of many traditional diets, including Chinese and Indian cuisine—in chapter 9. For now, it's enough to know that reaping the benefits of fermented foods is as easy as adding yogurt to your breakfast, a pickle to your sandwich, or a side of sauerkraut to your dinner.

Fats: Rebalance Your Ratios

The fat-free craze of the mid-1990s is long gone, but some of my patients have never quite gotten over fat phobia. Believe me, I understand. Back in the day, I myself succumbed to that unreasonable fear of dietary fat and hoovered countless boxes of fat-free cookies.

But nutritionists have extolled the benefits of healthy fats for decades now—and studies are revealing more discoveries every day. One is that we need a balance between omega-6 fatty acids and omega-3 fatty acids. Both are "essential"—our bodies can't make them, but we do need them for good health. However, we consume far too many omega-6s and far too few omega-3s. In fact, the typical American diet contains 14 to 25 times more omega-6s than omega-3s. That's a serious imbalance, largely due to the high amounts of processed foods and oils in the Western diet.

A 2012 commentary published in the journal *Environmental Health Perspectives* noted that an unhealthy diet actually makes you more vulnerable to pollution's negative health effects. To help manage these effects, it suggests changing the ratio of omega-6s and omega-3s in our diets. Specifically, eat fewer processed foods and more that are high in omega-3 fats, such as salmon, flax seeds, walnuts, and sardines. Rebalancing this ratio can help support immune response and cool inflammation.

So, our bodies—and guts—need the right kinds of fats, in the right amounts. The right kinds include avocados, olives, nuts, olive oil, coconut oil, avocado oil, and peanut oil. Ditto for ghee (clarified butter), a staple of

Indian cuisine. In Ayurvedic medicine, ghee is considered to stimulate and increase agni. These fats help regulate digestion and keep your cell membranes healthy and your gut lining intact.

The right amount? A drizzle here, a drizzle there, a few chunks of avocado on your salad, a handful of nuts as a snack. Studies show that even small amounts of healthy fats can slow digestion—helping you to feel satisfied for longer—and improve absorption of nutrients like vitamin D and vitamin E.

The fats to eat less of: saturated fats—found primarily in animal foods (bacon, cheese, red meat, milk)—and trans fats, found in fried foods like French fries and doughnuts, baked goods such as cookies and crackers, and stick margarine.

Grains: Go with Them

Having snuck into virtually every processed food in one form or another, grains are now a staple of the American diet. I frequently test my patients for gluten intolerance, and many can trace their digestive or other health problems to gluten-containing grains (wheat, barley, rye, and spelt). When they stop eating them for a time, their symptoms improve.

Why should this be so? Whole grains brim with fiber and nutrients. They've been linked with bacterial diversity in the gut. Nutritionally speaking, grains have a lot going for them.

However, celiac disease is four times more common now than it was sixty years ago. It's been suggested that its rise might be attributable to an increase in the gluten content of wheat—a result of modern breeding methods. A recent study published in *The Journal of Agricultural and Food Chemistry* disputed that theory.

So what's going on?

Well, we eat far more wheat- and gluten-containing grains than we used to, and *that* may account for the increase in celiac disease, and perhaps gluten sensitivity, according to the study. Further, food manufacturers use wheat gluten as an additive in tons of processed foods. While gluten doesn't pose problems for everyone, it is one of the most difficult proteins to digest. The overexposure to wheat, whole grains, and gluten wears down the gut lining, thereby triggering leaky gut and the conditions that result from it.

I suspect that another cause of the heightened sensitivity to gluten is the hybridization of wheat. In hybridization, scientists choose particular strains of a plant with desirable characteristics, then breed them. Because of this repeated breeding, modern wheat bears no resemblance to its "ancestors." The lack of variation of types of grain, or even types of wheat, has created a lack of probiotic diversity in our guts. They are exposed to the same bacteria over and over again, rather than the mix of bacteria our grandparents and great-grandparents got by eating seasonally or eating varied crops.

If you're not sensitive to wheat or whole grains, they are a valuable source of fiber, B vitamins, antioxidants, and trace minerals. But stick to the grains themselves, rather than boxed cereals or crackers. (See my "cardboard rule" on page 68.)

If you have digestive symptoms and cannot trace their source, the 21-Day Belly Fix can help solve the mystery. If it turns out that you are sensitive to gluten, then brown rice, quinoa, oats, millet, wild rice, and buckwheat are tasty and nutritious alternatives. Their carbohydrates will energize you, and their fiber will sweep toxins from your digestive tract.

Sugar: Limit or Eliminate Refined Sugar

Doughnuts for breakfast. A Snickers bar at the office. Ice cream after dinner. And sugary drinks—soda, fruit juices, coffee drinks, bottled teas—all day. At times, to me, the food supply seems like an ocean of sugar—and Americans are going under. It's estimated that the average American consumes 22 teaspoons of added sugars a day!

Why does sugar unbalance our gut stew? A large part of the reason: a gut beastie with a sweet tooth. Called *Candida albicans,* this common yeast lives on the sugars in our gut. And if you eat the typical Western diet, this yeast feasts! Our diets are simply too high in white sugar, high-fructose corn syrup, and foods made with refined grains, which act just like sugar in your body. Foods made with refined grains include sliced sandwich bread, white pasta, boxed baked goods (cookies, doughnuts, cakes), and salty snacks. White rice is a refined grain, too—it's had its nutritious germ and bran removed.

When a high-sugar diet creates an overgrowth of *C. albicans,* the result is a condition known as candidiasis. Common symptoms include abdominal pain, bloating after meals, constipation, and flatulence. Many patients also have other signs or symptoms: yeast infections, dry, flaky patches of skin, seborrhea in the scalp or an intensely itchy rash on the trunk and back.

Candida has significant health implications for both adults and children. Children with candida can develop ADD/ADHD, anxiety, bipolar disorder, allergies, eczema, and asthma, while adults typically develop reflux, depression, anxiety, and chronic sinusitis.

A high-sugar diet doesn't just disrupt your gut flora, however. It also wears down your gut lining and overburdens the liver. The American Heart Association has set strict limits for added-sugar consumption—6 teaspoons (24 grams) of added sugars per day for women, and 9 teaspoons (36 grams) for men. Typically, I limit my patients to 40 grams of sugar a day. Only 10 grams is from added sugars, the rest from carbohydrates and fruit.

Proteins: Pick the Right Ones for You

Protein is found in many different foods—beans and peas, tofu and tempeh, milk and cheese, fish and fowl, eggs and red meat. Protein-rich foods are a crucial part of any healthy diet, including the 21-Day Belly Fix. They're excellent sources of glutamine, the most abundant amino acid (building block of protein) in the body. One role of glutamine is to help protect the lining of the gastrointestinal tract. Protein contains additional amino acids and nutrients that help the gut hum along smoothly and balance neurotransmitters and hormones.

However, some people are sensitive to proteins, and that sensitivity can contribute to a leaky gut. I have found that patients with gut issues are

The Ultimate Probiotic

Unfortunate name, miraculous results. I'm talking about a fecal microbiota transplant (FMT), in which poop from a healthy person, teeming with billions of gut-friendly bacteria, is transplanted into the colon of someone with the severe bacterial infection *Clostridium difficile.*

The illness most commonly affects older people in hospitals or in long-term care facilities, typically after the use of antibiotics. Alarmingly, however, *C. difficile* infection is on the rise among young, healthy people who have not taken antibiotics. People who take medications to reduce stomach acid, including proton pump inhibitors (PPIs), are also at higher risk. In its severe form, *C. difficile* infection can cause bouts of watery diarrhea up to fifteen times a day, extreme abdominal cramping and pain, and kidney failure.

Nor does the infection always respond to antibiotics. In fact, taking antibiotics for long periods, as you might if you had the infection, wipes out much of the friendly gut bacteria that would normally help fight the bad bug.

In an FMT procedure, doctors take stool from a healthy donor, perhaps the size of a golf ball. They dilute it with saline, then flush it through a tube inserted into the sick person's colon, covering the colon lining with the icky-but-health-giving mix. Recipients typically feel better within days, as the healthy person's abundant and diverse gut bacteria wipe out *C. difficile* and recolonize the sick person's bowel with good gut bugs.

This procedure isn't some crazy, last-ditch measure, either. A 2013 study published in *The New England Journal of Medicine* found FMT significantly more effective in treating recurrent *C. difficile* infection than the antibiotic vancomycin. Of 16 study volunteers, 13 had resolution of their infection after just one poop infusion. That's an 81 percent success rate! A second treatment cured two others.

FMT also shows promise as a treatment for inflammatory bowel diseases such as Crohn's disease and ulcerative colitis. Typically, people with these conditions must take extremely powerful medications that suppress the immune system and cause other unpleasant side effects. How wonderful to think that, in the near future, they may be able to escape the misery of these illnesses—and the potent medications used to treat them—with a simple "poop transfusion."

often sensitive to a particular type of protein. We've discussed gluten, a protein in wheat, but the protein in dairy (casein) and proteins in certain meats and eggs can all potentially trigger food sensitivities and gut dysfunction.

If you have digestive issues, it's possible that you may have a sensitivity or intolerance to one or more proteins. My program will help you identify those foods so that you can get the protein your body needs and the glutamine your gut lining needs to heal.

Live by the "No-Cardboard Rule"

Just as algal blooms sicken oceans, processed food encourages a toxic microbial "bloom" in our guts that sickens *us*. Where to even begin with FINO? Well, for starters, it's fiber- and nutrient-poor. It's also "sterile"— assembled in manufacturing facilities that employ "clean rooms" to destroy the bad bacteria that can make us sick as well as the good bacteria that promote health. And then there's the evidence that a Western-style "FINO diet" promotes the low-grade, smoldering inflammation that ignites the spark of chronic disease. And its artificial flavorings and preservatives, such as monosodium glutamate, artificial sweeteners, and dyes, irritate the intestine and alter its pH, damaging or killing off friendly gut bugs.

I tell my patients that 90 percent of what they eat should be wrapped in its own skin—vegetables, fruits, whole grains (with or without gluten) that contain the bran. Just 10 percent or less of their food should come in cardboard boxes—or plastic wrappers or cans, for that matter.

I'm not saying that FINOs are permanently off the menu. (That's what the 10 percent is for!) But how about giving fermented foods a try?

They're definitely "processed," but this ancient food-preservation technique confers health, rather than illness. And how about cutting back on added and artificial sugars? That alone can make a significant positive difference in your health. Your weight, too—you need good gut bugs to help you digest and metabolize food. And a diet laden with the simple sugar fructose (found in both white sugar and high-fructose corn syrup) and artificial sweeteners may "Westernize" gut stew, a 2012 study published in the journal *Obesity Reviews* suggests. That is, gut bacteria may adapt to that glut of sugar and chemicals in ways that disrupt satiety signals and metabolism. Lose those, and it's possible that you may lose weight, too.

If you're used to eating with your eyes first, eating for your gut will take some getting used to. But the benefits to your body—as well as your mind and spirit—will be great. You'll have more energy than ever before, you'll have glowing skin, and you'll feel more vital and positive.

4. KNOW YOUR DIETS

Even if you want "no-diet weight loss," it's still smart to know what diets are out there, so that you can see how I developed the 21-Day Belly Fix. When I meet with a patient, "diet" plans—what works, which one he or she should be on—are one of the most common topics discussed. Not a day goes by that someone doesn't ask me about whether or not he or she should go paleo, gluten free, or dairy free or try out the latest plan touted on TV. Some of these "diets" I've never heard of—many patients have even been on their diet of choice for weeks or even months before they come to see me, still frustrated and unhappy about not losing weight, still having IBS or abdominal pain.

Chances are, if you've experienced unpleasant symptoms—gastrointestinal or other—you've wondered whether what you're eating could be causing your pain and discomfort. Perhaps you've had the same experience as so many of my patients, whose questions to their doctors about what to eat have turned up little valuable information. Since most doctors don't have much nutrition training, they tend not to be that comfortable giving out advice about diet. Many doctors don't even consider the role of food when giving advice to patients! They are trained to prescribe medication to get a person feeling well as soon as possible. Of course, there is a time and a place for medications, and we all can benefit from them. However, you cannot talk about gut health without discussing food first.

So, where do most people turn when they don't get the guidance they need from their doctor? Dr. Google, of course (it's okay—everyone does it!). When I typed "gut health diet" into my browser, it turned up more than 16,000,000 hits—many sites and blogs that praise with religious fervor the various diets that people adhere to. Confused yet?

Here's my general take on these diets: They're not magic. They all have their benefits and drawbacks and can be helpful when used in the right way by the right person.

Below, we'll set the record straight on the five diets I get the most questions about. And in the next section of the book, we'll move on to the 21-Day Belly Fix—a plan that pulls from the best of each of these five plans and merges them with conventional gastroenterology, Ayurvedic medicine, and Chinese medicine.

Paleo

OVERVIEW: Short for "Paleolithic Diet," this plan is based on the idea that the way we ate when we were hunter-gatherers is ideal for optimal health. Paleo dieters eat grassfed meat, fish and seafood, fruits and vegetables, eggs, nuts and seeds, and oils like olive, flaxseed, and coconut. As a result, this diet is high in protein (mainly from meat and seafood), low in carbohydrates (since grains are forbidden, the main sources of them are fruits and vegetables), and high in fiber (from all of that produce).

PROS: The focus is on fresh. You'll eat a "clean" diet without preservatives or other chemicals. You'll feel satisfied, thanks to the high doses of filling protein and fiber, and you'll get a ton of disease-fighting antioxidants through your high intake of fruits and vegetables.

CONS: It assumes that all grains are bad. Many people have trouble tolerating some grains but not others. For those who aren't sensitive to them, whole grains can be an extremely valuable source of energy—carbs are your brain's preferred energy source—as well as fiber, B vitamins, and more. Why throw out the baby with the bathwater?

Gluten Free

OVERVIEW: This diet excludes all foods that contain the protein gluten, which is found in wheat, barley, rye, spelt, and triticale. It is used to treat people with celiac disease, an autoimmune disorder in which exposure to gluten causes damage to the lining of the intestine, causing decreased absorption of nutrients that can lead to a long list of life-threatening complications. It is also used by people with non-celiac gluten sensitivity, a difficult-to-diagnose but more prevalent condition (the latest research suggests that at least six times more people have non-celiac gluten sensitivity than people who have celiac disease). People with non-celiac gluten sensitivity can experience a range of symptoms, but their bodies don't produce the same antibodies as someone with celiac disease, so they don't suffer the same intestinal damage.

PROS: If you have celiac disease or non-celiac gluten sensitivity, a gluten-free diet is 100 percent the right choice for you—the only choice, in fact (aside from something like Paleo or the Specific Carbohydrate Diet, which encompass gluten free). Doing so will give your intestines the opportunity to heal.

CONS: As gluten-free diets become more popular, it's becoming all too easy to eat a very unhealthy, yet completely gluten-free, diet. If your diet is comprised of gluten-free toaster pastries, cupcakes, BLTs, and fried mozzarella sticks, you're still flooding your gut with sugar and saturated fat. In addition, the gluten-free diet removes one possible offender, but it does nothing else to help heal your gut and replenish it with the nutrients and healthy bacteria it needs.

Specific Carbohydrate Diet

OVERVIEW: Initially intended for people with bowel diseases like Crohn's disease and ulcerative colitis, this diet was created in the 1950s by Dr. Sidney Haas and popularized by Elaine Gottschall, a biochemist and the mother of one of Haas's patients who later published a book on the diet called *Breaking the Vicious Cycle*. The SCD diet begins with an extremely limited introductory period and later expands to include a range of specified produce, meats, nuts, beans, and dairy. Hallmarks of the diet include both homemade yogurt and chicken soup.

PROS: Similar to the Paleo Diet, this plan excludes processed and sugary foods and gives you little choice but to eat a more natural, whole-foods diet. It takes time to transition through the different phases, allowing the gut some time to heal.

CONS: It's extremely restrictive—possibly overkill for someone who doesn't necessarily need it. The required homemade yogurt and chicken soup can be overwhelming for someone who's not comfortable in the kitchen.

GAPS (Gut and Psychology Syndrome) Diet

OVERVIEW: Based on the Specific Carbohydrate Diet, the GAPS diet was created by Dr. Natasha Campbell-McBride, a physician who coined the term "Gut and Psychology Syndrome" in recognition of the connection between the digestive system and the brain. Her book claims that GAPS can play a role in healing autoimmune issues, infertility, allergies, leaky gut, and more. This plan works in stages: The introduction diet includes healing broths, boiled meat and veggies, and gut-balancing probiotic ingredients, while the later phases introduce foods like fats (preferably from animal sources), vegetables, nuts, organ meat, and, eventually, some dairy. The plan completely eliminates grain foods, starchy vegetables, and sugars and also recommends specific dietary supplements as well as lifestyle changes.

PROS: The stages give the gut time to heal, and the slow reintroduction of foods gives you the opportunity to identify your trigger foods. It is also whole foods–based.

CONS: It's extremely restrictive—even more so than the Specific Carbohydrate Diet.

Low FODMAPs

OVERVIEW: Recommended for people with irritable bowel syndrome or those with symptoms such as cramping, bloating, gas, or diarrhea, this diet limits carbohydrates that are difficult to digest—specifically, ones that pull water into the intestinal tract and are fermented by bad bacteria when eaten in excess. FODMAPs is an acronym that stands for "**F**ermentable, **O**ligo-, **D**i-, **M**ono-saccharides **A**nd **P**olyols" and includes foods that contain high levels of fructose (like fruits and honey), lactose (found in dairy), fructans (found in wheat, garlic, onion), galactans (found in beans and lentils), and polyols (found in sugar alcohol sweeteners like xylitol and sorbitol, and stone fruits like apricots and plums).

PROS: It doesn't cut ingredients out, instead giving you a measured allowance of the offending foods each day. As a result, it encourages well-balanced eating.

CONS: It may not be enough for someone with a serious sensitivity to gluten, dairy, or grains, since it only limits these foods rather than eliminating them completely. Can also be a low-fiber diet, since it limits so many fiber-rich ingredients.

Now that you know what's out there, you'll see why my 21-Day Belly Fix makes sense. Rather than giving you one rigid set of foods you're allowed to eat, this plan starts slow, resting and soothing a depleted GI tract, plugging the holes in your leaky gut, repopulating it with healthy bacteria, and then carefully reintroducing foods, giving you the opportunity to identify the triggers that got you off track in the first place.

five

The 21-Day Belly Fix: Days 1–3

THE GUT AT REST

I see it in practice every day—overworked bellies, trying desperately to get a break. What with less-than-stellar food choices, alcohol, toxins, and more, the work of digestion can be rough and exhausting. Yes, it is true; even your belly needs a vacation. You may not be aware of it, but I can see it: The bloated belly, puffy face, excessive sweating, coated tongue, broken fingernails, and rashes (not to mention that stubborn last ten pounds) are all signs that it is now time to get out of the gutter.

Good gut health begins by resting the belly. Digesting and breaking down food can be a lot of work for a depleted GI system. Specific foods like wheat and dairy are often blamed for digestive issues, but in reality any food can be problematic if the entire GI system has been injured. Remember our players—the gut lining, the bacteria, the enzymes—have all been worn away by the work of too much digestion. Often called "detox-ification," gut rest is all about giving your system a temporary break from its main job.

The concept of gut rest is not new; in fact, it is as old as our earliest texts. In systems of medicine that are thousands of years old, like Chinese and Ayurvedic medicine, gut rest was mandatory for optimal health. What I am calling the gutter, they referred to as "ama" or "stagnation." Ayurvedic medicine says that as ama collects, it creates heat that rises from that stomach and literally sets the rest of the body on fire. Chinese medicine practitioners use the terms *stagnation* and *dampness* to describe an overburdened belly. They envisioned a gut stopped up with a sticky, immobile mass that cannot be eliminated, making the rest of the body sticky, puffy, and swollen.

On my three-day gut rest, we are eliminating ama, getting rid of dampness and stagnation, and giving the belly a well-deserved vacation. The focus is on foods and drinks that will provide energy but are easily processed, minimizing the work of the gut. I've included some easy-to-digest fruit for fiber, nutrients, and flavor but kept the sugar content low, including fruit sugars, since too much can be hard on the gut and possibly promote the growth of yeast in the intestinal tract. You'll be following the same plan for all three days (don't worry, there are some built-in menu options to keep it interesting). This combination of items is designed to give your body the fuel it needs to thrive without the burden of hard-to-digest ingredients. In fact, many of the foods and drinks included in the 3-day gut rest are digestion-promoting and will contribute to reviving the gut and getting all the players back on the right bases.

Now, in all honesty: The first few days are not easy. And let's be clear about one thing: In my plan, resting your gut is not the same as fasting. For these next three days, we'll remove all of the major gut health offenders so that your GI tract has a chance to begin the healing process. You will, however, still be taking in calories in the form of whole foods like vegetables, fruit, and healthy oils (the calorie counts for each day are likely lower than your needs; I recommend that you take a break from exercise and unnecessary exertion over these three days). It's possible to feel withdrawal symptoms like headache and irritability from eliminating caffeine, refined sugar, and high-fat foods from your diet; this is normal for a few days, so don't feel discouraged if you don't feel your best right away. If symptoms persist past the first week of the plan, talk with your doctor.

It is simple and easy-to-follow and can clean out excess ama and improve your agni (the "fire" that drives digestion and metabolism) in just three days.

HERE'S THE PLAN

When you first wake up:

Three easy steps will help you set the stage for a well-functioning gut all day long. Begin your morning with the following foods and beverages to correct the gut pH level, to increase digestive juices, and to stimulate gut motility. Why these three things?

- An acidic *gut pH* sets the stage for digestion. It's true—while antacids (medications that counter acid in the gut) are some of the most commonly used medications in the United States, the stomach is actually *supposed* to be acidic. The acidic environment serves to kill bacteria, break down proteins, and activate crucial enzymes and hormones needed for digestion. The pH of a healthy belly is around 1–3 when it's empty, rising to 4–5 after a meal.
- This pH differs from your overall body pH, which should not be acidic. In my practice, we will often use saliva or urine pH to determine where your overall pH lies. If your pH is under 6.8, you are acidic where you should not be—which means you probably don't have enough acid in your stomach.
- *Digestive juice* (or gastric juice) is a clear, acidic liquid secreted by the glands in the lining of the stomach. It's mainly made up of hydrochloric acid (of which the stomach produces roughly two liters per day), the digestive enzymes pepsin and rennin, and mucus. As hydrochloric acid creates an ideal environment, enzymes begin the process of breaking down proteins; mucus is there to help protect the lining of the stomach from its acidic contents. Producing an adequate amount of this gastric juice is crucial for getting digestion off to the right start.
- *Gut motility* is a fancy way of describing the controlled movements of the GI tract that help move food through the various steps of di-

gestion. Nerves and muscles within the GI tract control gut motility; their normal patterns can be affected by sleep habits, emotional stress, and the foods you eat, among other factors. Heartburn, constipation, abdominal distention, and diarrhea are some symptoms of gut motility dysfunction; proper gut motility creates the perfect setting in which food can be broken down, nutrients absorbed, and waste eliminated.

Next, you will find the steps to accomplishing these three goals.

Drink Apple Cider Vinegar

Apple cider vinegar is an old folk remedy that devotees have recommended for everything from hiccups to diabetes. Hippocrates, the "Father of Medicine," is reported to have prescribed it for a variety of ailments. I find that apple cider vinegar diluted in a bit of water can help start the day on the right foot when it comes to breaking down and processing food. In addition to being rich in digestion-promoting acetic acid, it also has antimicrobial properties. Remember, when acid supplies are low, the GI system doesn't extract the right nutrients from food, which it then has to work much harder in order to process. An apple cider vinegar cocktail first thing in the morning will end your all-night fast by priming your stomach for proper digestion. Don't worry too much about the flavor—it's not as sour as you'd expect; still, you will want to drink the diluted apple cider vinegar rather quickly.

HOW: Dilute one tablespoon of unfiltered apple cider vinegar in three tablespoons of water (you'll drink it in water, since straight vinegar can damage tooth enamel or hurt the tissues in your throat and mouth).

Sip a Cup of Warm Ginger Tea

Ginger has long been well known as a digestive aid, an idea now supported by scientific research. Ginger contains phenolic compounds like shogaols that stimulate bile production and increase stomach acids. Now that you've used apple cider vinegar to prime the pH of the stomach, ginger will help get things moving and increase your digestive juices. The spicy rhizome speeds up the movement of food from the stomach into the small intestine, which aids in the motility of the gut, according to research published in *The European Journal of Gastroenterology and Hepatology.*

HOW: While you sip your apple cider vinegar cocktail, steep one teabag of ginger tea in a six-ounce mug of boiling water for three minutes; drink tea immediately after the apple cider vinegar beverage. I often skip the tea bags and instead, toss some slices of ginger root into my teakettle and sip on the warm water with a teaspoon of honey throughout the day.

Eat Two Brown Rice Cakes with Coconut and Olive Oils

Use brown rice cakes for a bit of insoluble fiber to help move food (in its various broken-down states) through the digestive tract. The fat in coconut oil is mainly made up of medium-chain triglycerides, which are easily digested, as well as the saturated fatty acid lauric acid, which has antimicrobial properties. Rich in antibacterial phenolic compounds, olive oil has been found by scientists to combat eight strains of the type of bacteria that are linked to peptic ulcers and gastric cancer. This combination will soothe and balance the gut while gently stimulating motility, aiding it in elimination and detoxification.

HOW: Spread two brown rice cakes each with one teaspoon of coconut oil and one teaspoon of olive oil.

Now that you've activated gut function, your belly is ready to take in some nutrients and to contribute to that microbial brew we keep referring to.

You'll accomplish this by having a mid-morning **protein shake**. The fruits in the shake recipe I've provided below will introduce some pre- and probiotic bacteria, providing microbial diversity to help balance the gut (we'll talk a lot more about that in chapter 8). I've also included easy-to-digest protein in the form of hemp, pea, or rice protein powders. Protein powders are often used in smoothies, but many of my patients, especially those with weak GI systems, cannot tolerate protein powders that contain whey, soy, or egg. It's not uncommon for people to have an allergy or intolerance to these proteins. That's why I insist on hemp, pea, or rice protein, all of which contain easily digestible amino acids, providing nutrients but minimizing the work of the gut. I recommend using one of the following products: Metagenics UltraClear Sustain, Vega Protein Smoothie, or Alive! Ultra-Shake Pea Protein. Use one scoop of protein powder—about fifteen grams of protein worth, along with 1–2 servings of produce to power up your day.

Here are a few options:

Blueberry Pie

MAKES 1 SERVING

½ cup frozen unsweetened wild blueberries
Juice of ½ lemon
1 scoop vanilla protein powder
½ cup water
½ cup ice

Blend all ingredients until thoroughly combined.

Per serving: 180 calories, 15.41 g protein, 3.56 g fat (.31 saturated), 22.09 g carbohydrates, 9.15 g sugars, 8.2 g fiber, 131 mg sodium

Banana Chocolate

MAKES 1 SERVING

1 medium banana, frozen
1 scoop chocolate protein powder
1 cup water

Blend all ingredients until thoroughly combined, adding water until desired consistency is reached.

Per serving: 256 calories, 17.37 g protein, 5.35 g fat (.44 saturated), 39.61 g carbohydrates, 16.43 g sugars, 9.2 g fiber, 141 mg sodium

Berry Blast

MAKES 1 SERVING

1 cup unsweetened frozen strawberries
½ medium avocado
1 scoop plain protein powder
½ cup ice cubes
Water as needed

Blend all ingredients until thoroughly combined, adding water until desired consistency is reached.

Per serving: 289 calories, 16.97 g protein, 13.64 g fat (1.76 saturated), 15.45 g carbohydrates, 15.45 g sugars, 13.7 g fiber, 138 mg sodium

Vanilla Date

MAKES 1 SERVING

1 Medjool date, pit removed
½ medium banana, frozen
1 scoop vanilla protein powder
1 cup water

Blend all ingredients until thoroughly combined, adding water until desired consistency is reached.

Per serving: 254 calories, 16.07 g protein, 3.23 g fat (.37 saturated), 42.47 g carbohydrates, 25.17 g sugars, 9.10 g fiber, 131 mg sodium

Tropical Colada

MAKES 1 SERVING

½ cup frozen mango chunks
½ cup cubed pineapple

1 scoop tropical or plain flavored protein powder

½ cup ice cubes

⅓ cup water

Blend all ingredients until thoroughly combined.

Per serving: 214 calories, 16.13 g protein, 3.41 g fat (.38 saturated), 31.78 g carbohydrates, 21.40 g sugars, 8.5 g fiber, 132 mg sodium

For lunch, which should be 3–4 hours after your morning protein smoothie, have one of my **Green Juice Blends,** made from fruit, dark leafy greens, and other vegetables that are known to detoxify and be easy to digest. The juice recipes I've featured in this book are blended drinks rather than juiced ones. The reason: fiber. Fiber not only helps you feel satisfied, it also helps keep your digestive tract humming by removing waste from the colon and providing a substrate for beneficial bacteria in the intestine (many juice drinks are made by removing the valuable fiber from fruits and vegetables). My recipes also include cruciferous vegetables like kale and watercress, which help to activate phase 2 detoxification enzymes that help prevent cell damage and promote the removal of carcinogens, among other beneficial effects like decreasing inflammation. The combination of dark, leafy greens and blended cruciferous vegetables helps to clean up your liver, preventing you from having "dirty liver syndrome," as we discussed in chapter 2. You can make a big batch the night before and just pour it into a to-go mug. If you like, you can have a second serving mid-afternoon.

The Refreshing One

MAKES 1 SERVING

½ medium apple

½ medium ripe pear

1 medium cucumber

¾ cup chopped kale

½ lemon, seeds removed

Chop the apple, pear, and cucumber. Add all ingredients to blender and pulse, adding water to thin as needed.

Per serving: 173 calories, 4.71 g protein, 1.08 g fat (.45 saturated), 43.11 g carbohydrates, 25.07 g sugars, 8.4 g fiber, 27 mg sodium

The Savory One

MAKES 1 SERVING

3 leaves romaine lettuce

1 celery stalk

2 kale leaves

½ large apple

¼ lemon, seeds removed

½ teaspoon grated ginger

½ cup water

Chop the lettuce, celery, kale, and apple. Add ingredients to blender and pulse until combined.

Per serving: 89 calories, 3.08 g protein, .85 g fat (.17 saturated), 21.29 g carbohydrates, 19.63 g sugars, 5.4 g fiber, 53 mg sodium

The Spicy One

MAKES 1 SERVING

1 large apple

2 stalks celery

1 cup chopped watercress

1 cup water

Juice of ½ lemon

Chop the apple, celery, and watercress. Add ingredients to blender and pulse until combined.

Per serving: 117 calories, 1.88 g protein, .54 g fat (.1 saturated), 29.61 g carbohydrates, 21.04 g sugars, 6 g fiber, 80 mg sodium

The Minty One
MAKES 1 SERVING

½ medium pear
¼ medium cucumber
½ cup chopped kale
½ cup chopped spinach
Juice of ½ lemon
5 peppermint leaves
1 cup ice cubes

Chop the pear and cucumber. Add the kale, spinach, lemon, and mint leaves to a blender and increase speed until the mixture is liquid. Add a quarter-cup of ice and blend, increasing ice by quarter-cup increments until the desired consistency is reached.

Per serving: 81 calories, 2.35 g protein, .54 g fat (.14 saturated), 19.83 g carbohydrates, 10.3 g sugars, 3.9 g fiber, 27 mg sodium

The Sweet One
MAKES 1 SERVING

½ medium banana, peeled
1 small orange, peeled
1 cup chopped kale
¼ cup water
1 cup ice cubes

Chop the banana and orange in half, and add to blender along with the kale and water. Blend until liquid. Add a quarter-cup of ice and blend, increasing ice by quarter-cup increments until the desired consistency is reached.

Per serving: 155 calories, 4.78 g protein, 1.02 g fat (.15 saturated), 36.90 g carbohydrates, 20.63 g sugars, 7 g fiber, 27 mg sodium

For dinner, again at least 3–4 hours after your juice blend, you can have any combination of vegetables you like (except for white potatoes), as long as they are steamed or sautéed in olive oil or coconut oil (or a combination of the two). In Chinese and Ayurvedic medicine, those with stagnation and excess ama should eat food that is cooked, steamed, or sautéed. Raw food is considered tough on the gut. You can also use unlimited herbs like dried or fresh oregano, basil, parsley, rosemary, thyme, and sage as well as spices like cumin, ginger, cinnamon, nutmeg, and cloves. These vegetables will further liver detoxification and "cleanup" while also resting your gut.

Here are a few examples:

1 cup each broccoli, snow peas, sliced red pepper, steamed and sprinkled with juice of a half-lemon and 1 tablespoon olive oil

1 cup defrosted frozen butternut squash and 1 cup chopped kale sautéed in 1 tablespoon coconut oil with a pinch each of nutmeg and cinnamon

1 cup cauliflower and 1 cup chopped rainbow chard sautéed in 1 tablespoon olive oil with a pinch each of red pepper flakes and cumin

3 cups frozen Asian stir-fry mix, sautéed in 1 tablespoon coconut oil with 1 crushed clove of garlic and ½ teaspoon grated fresh ginger

Do you exercise more than half an hour a day? If so, your calorie needs are higher. Add a second protein shake to make sure your body is getting the fuel it needs.

At the end of three days of soothing, digestion-promoting, gut-supportive foods, you should notice less abdominal pain and decreased bloating. By the end of these three days, you will have worked to improve your intestinal pH, increase your digestive juices, activate digestive enzymes, and detoxify your liver—all while still eating. You will have also taught your stomach and digestive system to expect to be nourished. Notice that each meal is spaced three to four hours apart to allow an adequate amount of time for the work of digestion to take place. Make sure your drinks, including water, are not iced but at room temperature or warm. Sticking true to Ayurvedic and Chinese medicine theory about gut rest, try not eating or drinking (other than water) after 8–9 p.m. to allow your belly a ten- to twelve-hour fasting period. It is in this time that the gut rests and prepares for another day of digestive work.

PLAN OVERVIEW

Meal/time	Food
Early morning (upon waking; 6:00-7:30 a.m.)	Diluted apple cider vinegar Warm ginger tea 2 rice cakes each spread with 1-2 teaspoons each coconut oil and olive oil
Mid-morning (10:00 a.m.)	One protein shake (choose from one of the recipes above, or create your own using 1 scoop protein powder and 1-2 servings of produce)
Lunch (1:00 p.m.)	Green Juice Blend
Dinner (5:00-6:00 p.m.)	Vegetables steamed or sautéed in olive oil or coconut oil

CALORIES: 800–1,000, DEPENDING ON YOUR PROTEIN SHAKE, GREEN JUICE, AND DINNER CHOICES. GIVEN THE LOWER CALORIE COUNT, WE DO NOT RECOMMEND EXCESSIVE EXERCISE FOR THE FIRST THREE DAYS OF THE 21-DAY BELLY FIX. FOCUS INSTEAD ON YOGA, WALKING, OR STRETCHING, OR JUST TAKE A TOTAL BREAK!

SHOPPING LIST

Apple cider vinegar, unfiltered (like the ones made by Bragg Organic, Dynamic Health, or Spectrum Naturals)

Ginger tea (100% ginger like the ones made by Alvita or Triple Leaf Tea), dried ginger root, or fresh ginger root

Brown rice cakes (like the ones made by Lundberg Family Farms or Quaker)

Produce Picks

Wondering why I included the fruits and vegetables I did in this chapter? Here's an overview of just some of the reasons:

Food	Top nutrition benefits	Why it's part of the 21-Day Belly Fix
Wild blueberries	An excellent source of disease-fighting antioxidants; may help prevent memory loss associated with aging.	Wild blueberries have prebiotic potential and may help balance the gut microbiota, according to research from the University of Maine.
Banana	Their combination of potassium and fiber make them a heart-healthy food.	A good source of pectin, a soluble fiber that can help ease constipation. Bananas that are less ripe are a good source of resistant starch, which feeds healthy gut bacteria.
Lemon	The limonoids in this tart fruit are potent cancer fighters.	In Ayurveda, the lemon is thought to be a purifier that can help remove ama from the digestive tract.
Strawberries	Just one cup has more than 100 percent of your daily need for vitamin C, which is important for the immune system and helps improve skin texture.	Strawberries contain approximately 2 grams of fiber per serving and are considered a low-sugar fruit, with only 4 grams per serving. They are also high in ellagic acids and flavonoids, which makes them potent anti-inflammatories.
Avocado	Since it's a low-carbohydrate food that is high in fiber, it's a great food for promoting healthy blood sugar levels.	Avocados provide a range of anti-inflammatory nutrients like alpha-linolenic acid, phytosterols, and carotenoids.
Dates	Dates contain a symphony of blood pressure–lowering nutrients like calcium, magnesium, zinc, copper, and more.	Dates are high in soluble and insoluble fiber, often can ease constipation and have a laxative effect.

Mango	In addition to being a good source of fiber, one cup of mango also provides 35 percent of your daily need of vision-protecting vitamin A.	Mangoes are a good source of digestive enzymes, which help break down protein and process food.
Pineapple	In addition to being a good source of vitamin C, it's also an excellent source of the mineral manganese, which plays an important role in energy production.	Pineapples are rich in the digestive enzyme bromelain, which helps break down protein and can counter inflammation in the body.
Apple	The antioxidant quercetin, concentrated in the apple skin, plays a role in decreasing inflammation.	Apples are a good source of the soluble fiber pectin, which can help regulate bowel movements.
Pear	A top source of inflammation-busting flavanols in our diets (thanks in part to their high concentration of epicatechins).	A low-allergen food, pears are easily digested by most since few have sensitivities to it.
Cucumber	This low-calorie vegetable is an excellent source of hydration.	The fiber and water content in cucumbers help promote healthy digestion.
Kale	This cancer-fighting cruciferous vegetable also plays a role in both steps of the body's detoxification process.	A high concentration of fiber can help keep the contents of your digestive tract moving.
Romaine lettuce	An excellent source of bone-building vitamin K.	High in fiber to ease digestive health, romaine lettuce also helps build bile by removing bile salts from the colon.
Celery	Despite being low in calories, celery is a good source of disease-fighting polyphenol nutrients.	The pectin fiber in celery can help decrease inflammation in the gut.
Ginger	A source of potent anti-inflammatory compounds called gingerols.	In Ayurvedic medicine, ginger is believed to strengthen agni and prevent the buildup of ama.

Watercress	A rich source of bone-building vitamin K, watercress also provides sulfur-containing compounds that are potent cancer-fighters.	Research shows that watercress induces detoxification enzymes.
Spinach	Rich in the carotenoids lutein and zeaxanthin, which help prevent macular degeneration.	Spinach is high in magnesium, a mineral important in easing gut motility and preventing abdominal bloating. Spinach is also high in vitamin K, which bacteria in the gut help metabolize.
Peppermint	The oils in fresh mint have antimicrobial properties.	Mint is thought to relax the walls of the digestive tract and is often used as a remedy for irritable bowel syndrome.
Orange	An excellent source of blood pressure-lowering potassium and fiber.	Oranges are a high-fiber fruit, often aiding in constipation. For some, however, the acid in oranges may irritate IBS or reflux.

Coconut oil, virgin or unrefined (like the ones from Spectrum Naturals, Dr. Bronner's, or Nutiva)

Olive oil, extra virgin, first cold pressed (like the ones made by Olave, Colavita, or Spectrum Naturals)

Fruits (amounts will depend on which smoothies or drinks you plan to prepare): frozen unsweetened wild blueberries, bananas, avocado, dates, frozen mango chunks, pineapple, apples, lemon, pears

Vegetables (amounts will depend on which smoothies, drinks, or meals you plan to prepare): kale, spinach, watercress, cucumber, celery, frozen Asian stir-fry mix, frozen butternut squash, broccoli, red bell pepper, snow peas, rainbow chard, cauliflower

Protein powder (I recommend Vega One, Metagenics UltraClear Sustain, Alive Ultra-Shake Pea Protein)

Herbs/spices: fresh ginger, fresh peppermint, garlic

six

The 21-Day Belly Fix: Days 4–6

PLUG YOUR LEAKY GUT

Congratulations—you have made it through three days of successful gut rest. Hopefully by now, your pH is improving, your digestive enzymes are activated, and your liver is a little cleaner. These are all important pieces of the 21-Day Belly Fix. We are now ready to move on to rebuilding the lining of your GI tract and plugging a leaky gut.

Rebuilding your gut lining is essential. You want the gut to be porous enough to allow the nutrients from food to enter your bloodstream and power your body, but not so permeable that undigested proteins, fats, and minerals pass through the gut without getting absorbed. We have already seen how the delicate mesh of the intestinal wall can be affected by our food choices, the bacteria in our bellies, and the quantity of our digestive juices. A leaky gut triggers inflammation, setting the stage for the many chronic disease of today: cancer, diabetes, metabolic syndrome, and auto-immune disease, just to name a few. Controlling inflammation, taking in the right blend of amino acids (the building blocks of protein) and balancing your gut microbiology will heal your gut. We've begun this process with gut rest, and we will now continue the process by introducing foods

Losing Motivation?

Consider purchasing pH strips and start testing your morning saliva and urine pH. Your goal is a pH higher than 6.8; this would be a sign that your digestive system is no longer acidic and starting to hum along more smoothly.

to the belly that are likely to be easily digestible, non-irritating, and helpful in rebuilding an already weakened intestinal lining.

During these next three days you will build on the basic gut rest plan with a few additions (noted in bold). Now that you've given your system a break, you can begin to turn the motor back up slowly. You will continue to wait 3–4 hours between meals and to finish eating by 9 p.m., allowing for a 10- to 12-hour fast before breakfast.

Here's one important note as you begin to incorporate new foods back into your diet. Introduce each new food one at a time, paying careful attention to how you react. If you experience general pain, digestive issues like abdominal discomfort, bloating, or diarrhea upon reintroduction of any food on the 21-Day Belly Fix, stop and put that food back on your "avoid" list, removing it again for at least six weeks. Continue with the 21-Day Belly Fix plan, looking out for recurrence of these symptoms at each step.

Since the average daily calories increase to around 1,200–1,600 at this stage in the plan, you should feel more satisfied than you did over the first few days. Withdrawal symptoms are likely to disappear or at least diminish, and you should feel less bloating and abdominal pain. As a result of the added caloric intake, you should also feel an increase in your energy level.

Here's what you'll eat, day by day:

DAY 4

Early Morning

You'll remember that the goal of the morning routine is to correct the gut pH level, to increase digestive juices, and to stimulate gut motility. Doing so will help create an environment that is just right for healthy digestion.

Just like the first three days, you'll have:

Apple cider vinegar cocktail: One tablespoon of vinegar diluted in three tablespoons of water.

Warm ginger tea: One teaspoon of ginger tea steeped in a six-ounce mug of boiling water or one tablespoon of fresh ginger root boiled in four to six ounces of water.

Rice cakes spread with coconut and olive oils: Two brown rice cakes, both spread with a teaspoon each of coconut oil and olive oil.

Mid-Morning

Protein shake (recipes found on pages 79–81 in chapter 5)

Lunch

At your midday meal you'll add **one serving of kitchari or sticky rice**:

These are two easily digestible foods used to heal the gut in Ayurvedic and Chinese medicine. *Kitchari* means mixture, usually referring to a combination of two grains, typically rice and mung beans. In Ayurvedic and Chinese medicine, kitchari is considered a purifying food that is used to help cleanse the body. It provides easy-to-digest nourishment while allowing the body to rest and heal. Kitchari improves digestive fire or agni, balancing pitta and helping the body to eliminate ama, the stagnation we talked about throughout the book. The mung beans, soaked for at least three hours prior to cooking, are thought to clear toxins from the body. Preparing and eating kitchari is a routine part of detoxification rituals in

Ayurveda. Remember my patient with colon cancer? This ritual of weekly kitchari was what his Ayurvedic physician used to prescribe in India, until he came to the United States and embraced a Western diet.

In Chinese medicine, sticky rice (also known as glutinous rice) is thought to have a warming effect that coats and soothes the walls of the stomach. It is recommended for those with "yin" constitutions who don't have much heat energy in their bodies and typically feel cold or plagued by "damp heat," making the work of digestion difficult. Sticky rice is usually cooked for longer periods of time than traditional rice, but with extra water.

Both these systems include a fat: ghee, coconut oil, or olive oil to help cleanse the gut. Coconut oil, as we have discussed, contains the medium-chain triglycerides that are more easily absorbed by the digestive tract, improving gut motility and elimination, ultimately improving absorption of all the crucial nutrients in your food. There are also anecdotal reports that coconut oil will reduce candida in the gut.

Ghee or clarified butter has been used in Ayurveda for centuries. Ghee is made by bringing butter to a simmer and straining out the milk solids, which are thought to be high in lactose. What you're left with is a healthy fat that stimulates the production of stomach acid and speeds up metabolism, rather than slowing it down like butter or margarine (ghee is a good source of medium- and short-chain fatty acids, which is likely responsible). Ghee stimulates and increases agni and helps get rid of dampness or damp heat.

Olive oil slows digestion as well, helping you to feel satisfied for longer. It also supports the pancreas by regulating the release of insulin, preventing another modern-day plague, insulin resistance.

Confused about which one to use? Try alternating or rotating the different healthy digestive fats to find the one that best suits you. If you can tolerate all three, then have some fun switching them around to vary your nutritional dividends!

Here are the two recipes:

Dr. Taz's Kitchari

MAKES 4-6 SERVINGS

1 cup basmati rice, rinsed well

1 cup dry mung beans, soaked in water for 3 hours

4 cups water

2 teaspoons salt

1 teaspoon grated fresh ginger

1 tablespoon ghee or coconut oil

2 teaspoons turmeric

Mix ingredients in pressure cooker; keep under pressure for 6–7 minutes. If you don't have a pressure cooker, combine ingredients in a saucepan and bring to a boil. Reduce heat, cover, and simmer for approximately 45 minutes or until rice and mung beans are soft.

Dr. Taz's Sticky Rice

MAKES 4 SERVINGS

8 cups water

1 cup sticky or glutinous rice, rinsed well

½ teaspoon salt

4 quarter-inch slices of ginger

2 tablespoons olive oil or coconut oil

Bring water and rice to a boil. Reduce to simmer and add ginger and oil; cook for 30–40 minutes or until rice is ready to eat.

So today, your lunch will look like this:

Green Juice Blend (recipes found on pages 81–84)
Kitchari or sticky rice: 1 cup

Day 4 at a glance:

Meal/time	Food
Early morning (upon waking; 6:00–7:30 a.m.)	Diluted apple cider vinegar Warm ginger tea 2 rice cakes, each spread with 1–2 teaspoons coconut oil and olive oil
Mid-morning (10:00 a.m.)	One protein shake (choose from one of the recipes in chapter 5 or create your own using 1 scoop protein powder and 1–2 servings produce)
Lunch (1:00 p.m.)	Green Juice Blend 1 cup kitchari or sticky rice
Dinner (5:00–6:00 p.m.)	Vegetables steamed or sautéed in olive oil or coconut oil

CALORIES: 1,000–1,200

DAY 5

Today will look just like day 4, with the addition of bone broth soup, a common medicinal food used in cultures around the world from Africa to India to Korea to heal the sick, the elderly, and the very young, to your dinner. Not only is bone broth soup easily digestible, but it is also rich in gelatin, which attracts and holds liquids including digestive juices. The gelatin also heals the gut lining, while the many amino acids, including proline and glycine, are important for healing connective tissue; building DNA, RNA, and proteins; and reducing inflammation in the body. Bone broth soups are typically made of bones with a small amount of meat and allowed to simmer for long periods of time, sometimes up to twenty-four hours. This is to maximize the amount of minerals and nutrients that are leached from the bones. Having married into an Indian family, my in-laws worked hard to "revive" me after the birth of my first child by preparing their family's classic "mutton soup," made of small amounts of goat meat with lots of bones. I remember at the time looking at the bowl and seeing the layer of gelatin on top and wondering if this soup could in any way be good for me. Years later, I finally get it—this had been passed down over generations as the secret to healing the body after major life events, like illnesses or pregnancy.

Here are two recipes:

Chicken Bone Broth Soup

MAKES 10-12 SERVINGS

2–3 pounds of bony chicken parts (wings, necks, etc.)

4 quarts cool, filtered water

2 tablespoons apple cider vinegar

3 carrots, peeled

2 medium onions, chopped

3 celery stalks chopped

¼ cup chopped parsley

Note: Farm-raised, free-range chickens give the best results.

Place the chicken pieces in a large pot with water, vinegar, and all vegetables except parsley. Let it sit for 30 minutes. Over medium flame, bring to a vigorous boil. Skim off any scum that rises to the top; reduce heat and cover. Simmer for a minimum of 8 hours. For more flavorful stock, simmer longer. Add the parsley for the final 15–30 minutes.

As the soup cools, use a slotted spoon to remove any large chicken and vegetable pieces. Strain out the remaining pieces through a metal colander and pour the broth into one large bowl or several small glass bowls. Chill in your refrigerator, skimming off any fat that congeals at the top. Store the broth in the refrigerator or freezer, depending on how quickly you plan to use it.

Slow Cooker Beef Bone Broth

1 medium carrot, chopped

1 medium celery rib, chopped

1 small onion, chopped

Around 2 pounds of beef bones

1 bay leaf

2 tablespoons apple cider vinegar

4 quarts cold, filtered water

Place the carrots, celery, onion, beef bones, bay leaf, vinegar, and water in the bottom of a 6-quart slow cooker. Make sure the ingredients are submerged; if not, add more water. Pour in enough water to submerge all of the ingredients. Set the slow cooker to low and set for a minimum of 8–10 hours and cover with lid (the longer you cook your soup, the more nutrients will be extracted from the bones). When the time is up, strain the ingredients so you are left with a translucent brown broth. Refrigerate broth overnight so you can scrape off and discard some of the solidified fat from the top. Reheat on stove when you are ready to eat it.

Day 5 at a glance:

Meal/time	Food
Early morning (upon waking; 6:00–7:30 a.m.)	Diluted apple cider vinegar Warm ginger tea 2 rice cakes, each spread with 1–2 teaspoons coconut oil and olive oil
Mid-morning (10:00 a.m.)	One protein shake (choose from one of the recipes in chapter 5 or create your own using 1 scoop protein powder and 1–2 servings produce)
Lunch (1:00 p.m.)	Green Juice Blend 1–2 cups kitchari or sticky rice
Dinner (5:00–6:00 p.m.)	Vegetables steamed or sautéed in olive oil or coconut oil Bone broth soup

CALORIES: 1,300–1,500

DAY 6

Day 6 is similar to day 5, with the addition of some lean protein in the form of white-meat chicken or turkey or white fish. Any of the three options add muscle-building, satiating protein as well as the energizing and immune-boosting minerals iron and zinc; if you opt for fish you're also adding in anti-inflammatory, heart-healthy omega-3 fatty acids. Lean meat is easier to digest than fattier cuts of meat—those take longer to break down, which can lead to constipation. Lean meat and fish are also better for you in general. The American Heart Association recommends it, along with beans, over fattier meats as your main sources of protein in order to prevent cardiovascular disease.

You can add this protein serving to your lunch or dinner; I suggest having it with dinner to make that a more substantial meal.

Day 6 at a glance:

Meal/time	Food
Early morning (upon waking; 6:00–7:30 a.m.)	Diluted apple cider vinegar Warm ginger tea 2 rice cakes, each spread with 1–2 teaspoons coconut oil and olive oil
Mid-morning (10:00 a.m.)	One protein shake (choose from one of the recipes in chapter 5 or create your own using 1 scoop protein powder and 1–2 servings produce)
Lunch (1:00 p.m.)	Green Juice Blend Kitchari or sticky rice (1–2 cups)
Dinner (5:00–6:00 p.m.)	Vegetables steamed or sautéed in olive or coconut oil 4–5 ounces white meat chicken or turkey, or white fish like flounder or sole Bone broth soup

CALORIES: 1,430–1,630

Note: For vegetarian substitutes, see page 140.

Recipes for Dinner (Combining Protein and Vegetables)

Mexican Stir-Fry

MAKES 1 SERVING

2 teaspoons olive oil

Pinch of red pepper flakes

Pinch of cumin

4 ounces chicken breast, sliced

½ cup white button mushrooms, sliced

½ red bell pepper, sliced

½ green bell pepper, sliced
1 tablespoon chopped fresh cilantro

Heat oil in a medium saucepan. Add the red pepper flakes and cumin. Add chicken and sear for about one minute. Stir-fry for about 2 minutes, until mostly cooked. Add the remaining ingredients. Continue to stir-fry until the vegetables and chicken are fully cooked (about 5 minutes).

Herbed Turkey Breast and Sweet Potatoes

MAKES 1 SERVING

1 medium sweet potato
¼ teaspoon dried sage leaves
¼ teaspoon dried rosemary leaves
¼ teaspoon dried thyme leaves
1 4-ounce turkey breast cutlet
1½ teaspoon olive oil

Preheat oven to 425°F. Scrub the sweet potato thoroughly with a brush under running water. Pat dry and poke with a fork. Wrap sweet potato in aluminum foil and bake for 45–60 minutes or until tender. Meanwhile, in a small dish, combine the sage, rosemary, and thyme leaves. Using your fingers, press the mixture onto the turkey breast. In a medium sauté pan or cast-iron skillet, heat one teaspoon of olive oil. Place the turkey cutlet in a hot pan and cook until bottom side is browned. Flip and brown on the other side, until cutlet is cooked through. Serve turkey and sweet potato together on plate, topping sweet potato with olive oil.

Spinach Sautéed in Olive Oil with Sole Topped with Lemon

MAKES 1 SERVING

1½ teaspoons olive oil (½ teaspoons + 1 teaspoon)
1 5-ounce sole fillet

3 cups baby spinach

½ lemon

Preheat oven to 400°F. Place sole in a shallow baking dish; drizzle both sides with a half-teaspoon of olive oil. Bake for about 30 minutes, or until fish is cooked through and beginning to flake, around 15 minutes (will vary depending on the thickness of the fish). While fish is cooking, preheat a medium sauté pan with the remaining teaspoon of olive oil. Add the garlic and spinach and sauté until the spinach is cooked. Place on dish next to the fish. Squeeze the half-lemon over it.

Ratatouille-Topped Chicken Breast
MAKES 1 SERVING

1½ teaspoons olive oil (1 teaspoon + ½ teaspoon)

½ small onion, diced

1 garlic clove, minced

½ cup eggplant, diced

3 or more tablespoons water

Pinch of salt

½ cup zucchini, diced

⅓ cup red bell pepper, diced

¾ cup tomatoes, chopped

1 tablespoon tomato paste

1 tablespoon basil, chopped

1 4-ounce chicken breast

Heat one teaspoon of olive oil in a medium sauté pan over a medium flame. Add the onions, cooking until translucent, about 5 minutes. Add the garlic and cook for another minute. Add the eggplant, two tablespoons of water, and salt and sauté until soft, adding additional water one tablespoon at a time as pan dries out; about 3–5 minutes. Add the zucchini and red bell pepper and cook another 5 minutes. Add the tomato, basil, and tomato paste and mix, cooking for an additional 5 minutes.

While the vegetables are cooking, drizzle the chicken with the remaining half-teaspoon of oil and, using a grill pan or countertop grill, cook for around 5 minutes on either side or until cooked through. Place chicken breast on plate and top with ratatouille.

Note: To make this recipe vegetarian, eliminate the chicken, instead adding a half-cup of chickpeas when you add the tomatoes and basil.

Thanksgiving Dinner

MAKES 1 SERVING

1 small sweet potato

1½ cups sliced Brussels sprouts

2 teaspoons coconut oil (1 teaspoon + 1 teaspoon)

1 4-ounce turkey breast cutlet

Preheat oven to 425°F. Scrub the sweet potato thoroughly with a brush under running water. With a fork, poke holes in the sweet potato and wrap in aluminum foil. Bake until tender, about 45–60 minutes. At the same time, place the Brussels sprouts in a cast-iron pan or on a baking tray and toss with one teaspoon of coconut oil. Bake for about 25–30 minutes or until Brussels sprouts become browned, tossing every 10 minutes. In the meantime, heat a small skillet with the rest of the coconut oil. Cook the turkey breast cutlet on one side until browned, flip, and cook on other side until cooked through. Serve turkey, sweet potato, and Brussels sprouts together on a plate.

Steamed Artichoke with Baked Flounder

MAKES 1 SERVING

1 medium artichoke

1 5–6-ounce flounder fillet

2 teaspoons olive oil

Pinch of dried oregano

Preheat oven to 425°F. In a small pot, add water up about one inch and bring to a boil. Trim off the top inch of the artichoke and pull off any small leaves around the base. Place artichoke in water, bottom side up, and simmer with the lid on for about 20–30 minutes or until you can easily insert a fork into the base. While artichoke is simmering, place flounder in a shallow baking dish, drizzled with a half-teaspoon of olive oil. Bake until fish can be easily flaked with a fork and is cooked through, around 8 minutes (will vary depending on thickness). In a small bowl, sprinkle remaining olive oil with oregano as a dipping sauce for the artichoke. Drain artichoke and serve along with the flounder.

Baked Spaghetti Squash with Tomato Sauce and Chicken Breast

MAKES 1 SERVING

1 small spaghetti squash
1 4-ounce chicken breast
1 teaspoon olive oil
1 clove of garlic, crushed
½ cup canned tomatoes, diced
⅛ teaspoon oregano

Preheat oven to 375°F. Cut a small slice off one end of the squash lengthwise so you can rest it on a baking dish and poke holes in the top with a fork. Place the squash in the baking dish and roast for about 45 minutes or until a fork can easily puncture the skin. Using a grill pan or countertop grill, cook the chicken breast until cooked through, about 5 minutes on each side. While the chicken breast is cooking, heat the olive oil in a small pan over medium heat. Add the garlic, tomatoes, and oregano and cook for about 5 minutes. When the spaghetti squash is ready, remove strands from the skin, place in a large bowl, and top with the tomato mixture and grilled chicken breast.

Turkey with Braised Root Vegetables

MAKES 1 SERVING

2 large carrots

1 large parsnip

1 small celery root

1½ teaspoons olive oil (1 teaspoon + ½ teaspoon)

½ cup water

½ teaspoon chopped fresh parsley

1 4-ounce turkey breast cutlet

Scrub the carrots, parsnips, and celery root and chop into bite-size pieces. Heat 1 teaspoon of oil in a sauté pan over medium flame. Add vegetables and sauté for about 5 minutes or until lightly browned. Add water and bring to a boil. Reduce to a simmer, cover pan, and cook until vegetables soften (around 15–20 minutes), removing the lid and adding parsley for the last minute or so. As vegetables are cooking, heat a small skillet with the rest of the olive oil. Cook the turkey breast cutlet on one side until browned, flip, and cook on other side until cooked through. Serve turkey and root vegetables together on plate.

Broiled Ginger Halibut with Mashed Turnips

MAKES 1 SERVING

2 cups turnips, diced into 1-inch cubes

1 5-ounce halibut fillet

1 clove garlic, chopped

¼ teaspoon grated fresh ginger

½ teaspoon olive oil

½ teaspoon coconut oil

1 teaspoon chopped cilantro

Bring a medium pot of water to a boil over a high heat. Add turnips and cook until tender, 20–30 minutes. In the meantime, line a broiler pan with foil and preheat in broiler for 5 minutes. Remove the pan from the oven and place the fish in the center, sprinkling with garlic, ginger, and olive oil. Return to broiler and cook until fish is just cooked through, around 8–10 minutes. Place on serving plate. When turnips are fork-tender, remove from heat and drain water thoroughly. Return turnips to pot and add the coconut oil and cilantro. Blend using a potato masher until relatively smooth. Serve on plate beside halibut.

Mexican Veggie Bowl

MAKES 1 SERVING

1 teaspoon olive oil
½ cup chopped zucchini
½ cup chopped carrots
½ cup black beans, rinsed and drained
¼ cup prepared salsa
¼ lime

In a small sauté pan, preheat olive oil over a medium flame. Add the zucchini and carrots and sauté until softened, about 5–7 minutes. Drain off any remaining liquid. Place in a large bowl and top with black beans and salsa; squeeze with lime.

PLAN OVERVIEW

Day 1–3 Total calories: 800–1,000	*Breakfast:* Diluted apple cider vinegar Warm ginger tea 2 rice cakes, each spread with 1–2 teaspoons coconut oil and olive oil *Mid-Morning:* One protein shake *Lunch:* Green Juice Blend *Dinner:* Vegetables steamed or sautéed in olive oil or coconut oil

Supplement Your Day

Now that your gut has taken it easy for nearly a week, today you'll also add in several supplements to support gut healing. While I often use supplements in my practice, I have to be very careful with recommending supplements to my patients with damaged guts. Over-supplementation can also be hard on the belly. But after a few days of gut rest, we have prepped the belly to handle the following supplements:

Glutamine. Glutamine might be one of my favorite remedies for the gut. I have lost count of the number of patients that have solved their belly issues by starting glutamine. As the most abundant amino acid (building block of protein) in the body, one of glutamine's roles is to help protect the lining of the gastrointestinal tract, also known as the mucosa. While under typical circumstances the body can produce enough glutamine, the introduction of stress and infections can cause the body to need more glutamine than it is able to make. People with irritable bowel disease, ulcerative colitis, and Crohn's disease, for example, lack an adequate amount of glutamine. Animal and human research both suggest that supplementing with glutamine may help repair damaged gastrointestinal mucosa.

Begin by taking approximately 500 mg of glutamine initially and then increase to 2–3 grams of glutamine within two weeks. I prefer glutamine for my gut patients in the form of a powder rather than a pill, since it is easier for the belly to absorb.

Aloe vera juice. This juice, extracted from the same plant you use to soothe sunburns, may also help settle your stomach. Aloe vera juice may help regulate gastrointestinal pH while helping to balance microorganisms in the gut. One recent study published in the Italian journal *Acta Bio Medica* found that aloe vera juice at certain concentrations promoted the growth of healthy bacteria. Add 1–2 ounces of aloe vera juice daily.

Digestive enzymes. These proteins, typically produced by the pancreas, stimulate chemical changes that facilitate digestion. The pancreas produces three types of enzymes—proteolytic enzymes break protein down into amino acids, lipases help turn fat into its smaller building blocks, and amylases help break carbohydrates into simple sugars. If you have lactose intolerance, you may have tried taking the digestive enzyme lactase in the form of a pill called Lactaid to help you digest dairy products comfortably. This will help to digest the carbohydrate lactose in dairy but will not help with the proteins (typically casein and whey). In my experience, I find that taking digestive enzymes like Creon (a prescription drug) or over-the-counter digestive enzymes that contain protease, amylase, or lipase digest the proteins, carbohydrates, and fats, respectively. These enzymes serve an important role in helping people with reflux, abdominal pain, and bloating.

Supplements to add, starting today: Glutamine powder (easier to digest than pills; 500 mg once per day between meals); aloe vera juice (1–2 ounces, once per day); digestive enzymes (at least once per day with your heaviest meal or any other meal you need help with)

Day 4 Total calories: 1,000–1,200	*Breakfast:* Diluted apple cider vinegar Warm ginger tea 2 rice cakes, each spread with 1–2 teaspoons coconut and olive oils
	Mid-Morning: One protein shake
	Lunch: Green Juice Blend Kitchari or sticky rice
	Dinner: Vegetables steamed or sautéed in olive or coconut oil

Day 5
 	
Total calories: 1,300–1,430
	Breakfast:
	Diluted apple cider vinegar
	Warm ginger tea
	1 rice cake spread with 1–2 teaspoons coconut oil and
	    olive oil
	
	Mid-Morning:
	One protein shake
	
	Lunch:
	Green Juice Blend
	Kitchari or sticky rice
	
	Dinner:
	Vegetables steamed or sautéed in olive oil or coconut
	    oil
	Bone broth soup

Day 6
 	
Total calories: 1,430–1,600
	Breakfast:
	Diluted apple cider vinegar
	Warm ginger tea
	1 rice cake spread with 1–2 teaspoons coconut oil and
	    olive oil
	
	Mid-Morning:
	One protein shake
	
	Lunch:
	Green Juice Blend
	Kitchari or sticky rice
	
	Supplements:
	Glutamine powder
	Aloe vera juice
	
	Dinner:
	Digestive enzymes
	Vegetables steamed or sautéed in olive oil or coconut
	    oil
	Bone broth soup
	4–5 ounces white meat chicken or turkey, or white fish
	    like flounder or sole

Days 4–6 average between 1,200 and 1,600 calories per day. This calorie amount, while variable, is a good range for most people. Dropping below 1,200 calories for extended periods can lower your metabolic rate, while going over 1,600 kcal can be too much food for some people. If you find you are needing to adjust calories in either direction, consider lowering or increasing the serving size of any of the foods. If you are very physically active, increase calories, using your protein shakes or lean protein with dinner.

Keeping a Symptom Diary

I find it can be helpful to keep a diet journal that includes room to write down not just what you're eating but also how you're feeling. The journal is valuable for two reasons: (1) It helps keep you honest, so you'll eat only the foods that are recommended on the plan. (2) When used in hindsight, it can help you pinpoint what symptoms may be related to a specific food you've eaten. Track using an old-fashioned notebook or a smartphone app like mySymptoms Food and Symptom Tracker.

Here's a sample diary you can use:

Time	Foods eaten	Symptoms
Early morning		
Mid-morning		
Early afternoon		
Mid-afternoon		
Early evening		
Late evening		

seven

The 21-Day Belly Fix:
Days 7–10

BUILD YOUR BACTERIA

Back in chapter 4, we talked about how having the right balance of "bugs" in the gut is critical to disease prevention. Good bacteria help us digest food, detoxify chemicals and hormones, prevent inflammation, and protect us from the bad bacteria that can make us sick. The more diverse the gut flora, the better.

In the first six days of this plan you've detoxed your diet, breaking the habit of eating processed and difficult-to-digest foods that can alter your gut microbiology. You have also detoxed your liver and lowered your load of yeast by lowering your intake of sugar and grain. You've eliminated those ingredients which, when eaten over and over again, can trigger inflammation that can set the stage for a leaky gut. To keep you moving on the path toward good gut health, this chapter will focus on adding foods and supplements that will help equip your gut with the microbes it needs to thrive, providing a variety of bacteria to the belly.

At this stage of the plan, you should feel lighter and more comfortable than you did before. Any digestive symptoms you'd been experiencing prior to beginning the 21-Day Belly Fix have likely subsided. You're taking in enough energy to keep your body adequately fueled without unnecessarily weighing your body down with excess calories (and if you feel as if you're not eating enough, it's okay to increase serving sizes moderately so that you feel satisfied). And the probiotic and prebiotic foods and supplements you'll be adding in at this stage will add to your sense of well-being as they repopulate the gut with the balance of microbes it needs to stay healthy, helping your body fight off infection and break down carbohydrates, among other functions.

Here's how you'll get there:

DAY 7

Today you're going to help bring the bacteria in your gut back into balance by adding one serving of a fermented food to one of your meals.

Why fermented food? The process of fermentation has been around since prehistoric times as a means of preserving and extending the life of perishable items. It is defined as "the conversion of carbohydrates to alcohols and carbon dioxide or organic acids using yeast, bacteria, or a combination thereof, under anaerobic conditions." You may be thinking, "Who on earth would want to eat that?" However, here are just a few of the fermented foods that you may already enjoy: yogurt, kefir, sour cream, pickles, sauerkraut, soy sauce, sourdough bread, beer, and wine.

Many of these foods were traditionally made using an "any of" culture that would begin the fermentation process, after which they would be allowed to sit and attract bacteria present in the natural environment. Even bread, a hundred years ago, was made at home and allowed to rise for days and weeks on end, growing and fermenting a vast array of bacteria. You may have read about bread makers today that do ferment their products; some have even found that people who are sensitive to gluten or grains in general can tolerate it, as long as the bread has been fermented!

Since all fermented foods are not created equal, I recommend adding one serving of any of the following foods per day at this stage.

Coconut milk yogurt or kefir. This is sometimes referred to as "cultured coconut milk." Since we haven't yet reintroduced dairy, as it is tough for many to digest and is considered an inflammatory food, I recommend a nondairy cultured food like coconut milk yogurt or kefir. It's produced very much the same way that dairy yogurts and kefirs are made, with several strains of healthy bacteria. Look for an unsweetened product to avoid taxing your stomach with unnecessary sugar, sugar derivatives, or preservatives.

Serving size: *One six-ounce carton of yogurt or a half-cup of kefir*

Sauerkraut. Directly translated as "sour cabbage" in German, sauerkraut is traditionally finely cut cabbage that has been lacto-fermented using nothing but salt, water, and the healthy bacteria that is naturally on the surface of the cabbage. Lacto-fermentation works because harmful bacteria don't like salt, while beneficial bacteria can tolerate it just fine. Submerging vegetables like cabbage in a salty brine creates an environment that limits bad bacteria but allows the good lactobacillus bacteria to thrive. The lactobacilli convert the carbohydrates in the cabbage to lactic acid, which preserves the vegetable and gives sauerkraut its characteristic vinegary flavor. When you buy sauerkraut, be sure to look for one that hasn't been pasteurized—the high temperatures used in that process kill off the beneficial bacteria. Many refrigerated brands have not been pasteurized; check with the individual companies to be sure. Of course, you simply make your own; for my recipe, see page 115.

Serving size: *a half-cup*

Kimchi. The traditional Korean side dish is made with vegetables like napa cabbage and daikon radish as well as garlic, salt, vinegar, and chili peppers. Similar to sauerkraut, the lactobacilli in kimchi help with digestion and may even prevent the growth of yeast infections. It's also thought to be a potent cancer fighter. To gain the maximum benefits, look for a brand that is refrigerated or make your own (for a basic recipe, see page 116).

Serving size: *a half-cup*

Tempeh. Made from fermented soybeans, this protein-rich meat stand-in retains many of the same nutrients found in whole soybeans, since it's minimally processed (at least in comparison with its soy cousin tofu, which goes through many steps of production before landing in your stir-fry). Tempeh is typically kept in the refrigerated dairy case of the supermarket, in a cake-like form packed in a tightly fitted plastic wrapper. Its mild nutty flavor works well in curries and stir fries as well as marinated and baked or roasted (you'll often find strips of tempeh seasoned and used as a stand-in for bacon in vegan BLT sandwiches). Try my tempeh dipping sticks (recipe on page 118) paired with one of my miso-based sauces (more on miso below)—you can also cut the pieces smaller or crumble them and use to top any dish.

Serving size: *Four ounces or about half a block of store-bought tempeh*

Miso paste. Not to be confused with the sushi bar staple miso *soup,* miso paste is a traditional Japanese seasoning made from mashed soybeans, salt, and a mold starter; the miso soup you sipped before that sushi dinner is made with miso paste, but the two are not interchangeable. In addition to its beneficial bacteria, miso paste is also a good source of disease-fighting antioxidants as well as digestive enzymes that help protect the stomach lining. Research has linked regular consumption of miso with decreased risk of gastric cancer, ulcers, and breast cancer. You will find various categories of miso paste (the most common varieties are white or red) in plastic tubs in the refrigerated section of health food stores, Asian markets, and conventional grocery stores with a good selection of international foods.

Serving size: *One tablespoon*

Kombucha. This fermented tea drink has become trendy in the last few years, but it is anything but new—it's thought to have originated in ancient China. Various forms of similar fermented tea drinks exist in many different cultures. While kombucha is probably not the cure-all devotees claim it to be, it can be a good source of probiotic bacteria, but adding some to your diet can help balance your gut.

Serving size: *a half-cup*

Starting today, add one serving of the above foods to any meal. I recommend adding a serving of coconut milk yogurt or kefir to breakfast or a serving of tempeh, sauerkraut, or kimchi to your lunch or dinner. Or you can use one of my miso sauce (see page 117) or dressing recipes (see page 118) on your vegetables at dinnertime. At this stage you'll also *remove* one of the rice cakes spread with coconut and olive oils from your breakfast, since you're now getting plenty of food throughout the day.

Day 7 overview:

Meal/time	Food
Early morning (upon waking; 6:00–7:30 a.m.)	Diluted apple cider vinegar Warm ginger tea 1 rice cake spread with 1–2 teaspoons coconut oil and olive oil
Mid-morning (10:00 a.m.)	One protein shake (choose from one of the recipes in chapter 6 or create your own using 1 scoop protein powder and 1–2 servings produce)
Lunch (1:00 p.m.)	Green Juice Blend Kitchari or sticky rice **Coconut yogurt/kefir, tempeh, sauerkraut, kimchi, or kombucha**
Dinner (5:00–6:00 p.m.)	Vegetables steamed or sautéed in olive oil or coconut oil **(or you can use a miso-based sauce to help meet your probioitic requirement)** 4–5 ounces white meat chicken or turkey, or white fish like flounder or sole Bone broth soup

| Supplements | Glutamine powder (500 mg, once per day between meals); aloe vera juice (1–2 ounces, once per day); digestive enzymes (at least once per day with your heaviest meal or any other meal you need help with) |

CALORIES: ABOUT 1,600

DAY 8

Now that you've upped your game with foods that contain healthy bacteria, we're going to take it a step further and add in a probiotic supplement. The reason: Since bacteria are living organisms whose survival depends on many factors, including temperature and pH, it's impossible to guarantee the level of probiotics you'll be getting through food. Probiotics levels in pills are also variable; however, including a reputable supplement each day on top of the food you're already eating will help ensure you get a valuable dose of the healthy bacteria.

When you're looking to buy a probiotic supplement, look for brands that have at least 20 billion cfu (colony forming units—that's the measure of a probiotic's strength) and at least 4–5 different strains of bacteria. In my practice, we mainly use Ortho Biotic Floraboost; I also recommend the prescription-grade probiotic VSL#3 for my patients with inflammatory bowel disease or those who need an extra boost. The higher the cfu count, the less need there is for refrigeration (unless the product specifies). I also recommend rotating the probiotic brand you use every six weeks to keep diversifying the microbes in your gut.

Day 8 overview:

Meal/time	Food
Early morning (upon waking; 6:00–7:30 a.m.)	Diluted apple cider vinegar Warm ginger tea 1 rice cake spread with 1–2 teaspoons coconut oil and olive oil
Mid-morning (10:00 a.m.)	One protein shake (choose from one of the recipes in chapter 6 or create your own using 1 scoop protein powder and 1–2 servings produce)

Lunch (1:00 p.m.)	Green Juice Blend Kitchari or sticky rice Coconut yogurt/kefir, tempeh, sauerkraut, kimchi, or kombucha
Dinner (5:00–6:00 p.m.)	Vegetables steamed or sautéed in olive oil or coconut oil (or you can use a miso-based sauce to help meet your probioitic requirement) 4–5 ounces white meat chicken or turkey, or white fish like flounder or sole Bone broth soup
Supplements	Glutamine powder (500 mg, once per day between meals) Aloe vera juice (1–2 ounces, once per day) Digestive enzymes (at least once per day with your heaviest meal or any other meal you need help with) **One probiotic supplement (at least 500 cfu).**

CALORIES: ABOUT 1,600

DAY 9

Healthy bacteria need to eat too. Today you'll begin supplementing with inulin, a prebiotic (a form of dietary fiber) that the healthy bacteria in your belly feed on, and eating at least one serving of prebiotic foods, like banana, garlic, onions, Jerusalem artichoke (see the recipe on page 119), wild blueberries, or chicory root. (With a deep, dark flavor, roasted chicory root is often used as a coffee substitute for those who cannot drink caffeine. Simply place one teaspoon in a tea infuser and steep in hot water for 7–10 minutes.)

Inulin supplements aren't as popular as probiotics. There's a brand of inulin powder called Prebiotin that you can order online. Look for this or another powdered brand. Try one dose for a few days; if you tolerate it well, slowly increase the dosage every few days until you're up to one scoop.

Day 9 overview:

Meal/time	Food
Early morning (upon waking; 6:00–7:30 a.m.)	Diluted apple cider vinegar Warm ginger tea 1 rice cake spread with 1–2 teaspoons coconut oil and olive oil
Mid-morning (10:00 a.m.)	One protein shake (choose from one of the recipes in chapter 5 or create your own using 1 scoop protein powder and 1–2 servings produce); **choose a shake that includes banana or wild blueberries for additional prebiotic fiber, or add onions and/or garlic to dinner.**
Lunch (1:00 p.m.)	Green Juice Blend Kitchari or sticky rice or fermented rice Coconut yogurt/kefir, tempeh, sauerkraut, kimchi, or kombucha
Dinner (5:00–6:00 p.m.)	Vegetables steamed or sautéed in olive or coconut oil (or you can use a miso-based sauce to help meet your probioitic requirement) 4–5 ounces white meat chicken or turkey, or white fish like flounder or sole Bone broth soup
Supplements	Glutamine powder (500 mg, once per day between meals) Aloe vera juice (1–2 ounces, once per day) Digestive enzymes (at least once per day with your heaviest meal or any other meal you need help with) One probiotic supplement (at least 500 cfu); one scoop prebiotic powder added to mid-morning shake

CALORIES: ABOUT 1,600

RECIPES

Sauerkraut

MAKES 6–8 SERVINGS

1 medium head of green or red cabbage

1½ tablespoons sea or kosher salt

Supplies: Cutting board, large knife, large mixing bowl, large mason jar, cheesecloth, rubber band, fork.

Give all of your supplies (including your hands) a good cleaning—you want the bacteria on the surface of the cabbage to not have to compete with any other microbes. Remove the limp outer leaves of the cabbage and set aside. Chop the cabbage, removing the tough inner core, and shred the rest. Transfer to the bowl and sprinkle with salt. Massage the salt into the shredded cabbage using your hands until the cabbage becomes watery. Using your hands, pack the cabbage into the mason jar. Pour the remaining liquid on top of the shredded cabbage. Use one of the outer leaves of the cabbage to weigh down the shredded cabbage to ensure that it stays submerged in its liquid. Cover the mouth of the jar with cheesecloth and secure with a rubber band. Every few hours, remove the cheesecloth and press the cabbage down with a fork so that it is even more submerged in the liquid. Return cheesecloth and allow to ferment in a cool, dark place for three or more days. Once you like the flavor of the sauerkraut, replace the cheesecloth with a lid and store it in the refrigerator for up to two months.

Kimchi

MAKES 6-8 SERVINGS

1 Napa cabbage (around 2 pounds)
¼ cup sea or kosher salt
1 teaspoon sugar
2 teaspoons grated ginger
1 tablespoon minced garlic (about 6 cloves)
3–4 tablespoons spring water or filtered water
1–5 tablespoons Korean red pepper flakes, also called kochugaru, depending on your desire/tolerance for heat
4 scallions, trimmed and cut into 1-inch pieces
8 ounces daikon, peeled and cut into matchsticks

Clean your hands and supplies well. Cut the cabbage into four equal quarters and remove the tough inner core. Cut each quarter across, into

2-inch-wide strips. Place the cabbage in a large bowl and sprinkle with salt. Use your hands to massage the salt into the cabbage until it begins to turn soft. Submerge the cabbage in the spring or filtered water and let stand for 1–2 hours, turning it once halfway through. Rinse the cabbage well under cold water three times. Pour it into a colander and drain it for 15–30 minutes. In the meantime, clean the bowl you used for salting and set it aside for later. In a small bowl, combine the sugar, ginger, garlic, 3 to 4 tablespoons of spring or filtered water, and the Korean red pepper flakes and mix to form a smooth paste. Squeeze any excess water from the cabbage and put it back into the large bowl. Add the scallions, daikon, and paste to the bowl, mixing everything together until the vegetables are evenly mixed and thoroughly coated with the paste (use your hands—gloves optional). Pack the kimchi into a large glass jar with a tight-fitting lid, pushing the cabbage down so that brine covers the vegetables. Leaving one inch empty at the top, seal the jar with the lid. Let the jar stand at room temperature for 5–14 days on a plate or in a bowl, since some of the brine can seep out of the jar. Check on the kimchi once a day, pressing down on the vegetables to ensure that they remain submerged in brine. Refrigerate before eating and keep for up to a month.

Ginger Miso Stir-Fry Sauce

MAKES 4–6 SERVINGS

½ cup hot water
¼ cup white miso
1 tablespoon toasted sesame oil
2 teaspoons grated fresh ginger
1 clove garlic, crushed and minced

Whisk the ingredients together in a small bowl. Add to stir-fried vegetables for the last 1–2 minutes of cooking.

Coconut Miso Stir-Fry Sauce

MAKES 4-6 SERVINGS

¼ cup white miso
¼ cup hot water
½ cup canned coconut milk
3 tablespoons chopped cilantro

Dissolve miso in hot water. Whisk in coconut milk and add cilantro. Add to stir-fried vegetables for the last 1–2 minutes of cooking.

Lemony Miso Tahini Dressing

MAKES 4-6 SERVINGS

¼ cup white miso
¼ cup tahini
Juice of ½ lemon
Hot water

Whisk together ingredients, adding water until the desired consistency is achieved. Use to dress steamed vegetables or as a dipping sauce for vegetables (you might want to leave it a bit thicker for this purpose).

Tempeh Dipping Sticks

MAKES 2 SERVINGS

1 block tempeh
2 tablespoons coconut oil

Preheat oven to 375°F. Slice block of tempeh into finger-length strips about a quarter-inch thick. Grease a cast-iron pan or baking sheet with one tablespoon of coconut oil. Arrange tempeh neatly and bake for about 15–20 minutes or until the bottom side begins to form a crust. Flip pieces with a spatula, add the other tablespoon of coconut oil, and cook another 15–20 minutes or until browned on both sides.

Baked Jerusalem Artichokes

MAKES 4-6 SERVINGS

2 pounds Jerusalem artichokes
2 tablespoons olive oil

Preheat oven to 375°F. Scrub Jerusalem artichokes and cut into one-inch cubes. Spread onto baking sheet and drizzle with olive oil, tossing to distribute. Roast for about 45 minutes or until golden brown, tossing every 5–10 minutes.

SHOPPING LIST

Coconut milk yogurt or kefir (look for an unsweetened one)
Sauerkraut (look for an unpasteurized brand like Bubbies, Great Lakes Kraut, or Karthein's Organic, or ingredients to make your own).
Tempeh (look for an organic brand like LightLife, WestSoy, or Soy-Boy)
Kimchi (or ingredients to make your own)
Miso Paste (red, white, or yellow, made by brands like South River Miso Company)
Probiotic supplement (look for one with at least 20 billion cfu, like Ortho Biotic Floraboost)
Inulin supplement: Powdered form; 500 mg per serving
Probiotic foods: Banana, garlic, onion, Jerusalem artichokes, wild blueberries, chicory root
Tahini
Coconut milk
Lemon
Cilantro

Ginger
Garlic
Sesame oil

OUTSIDE RESOURCES

Fermentation

Patrick McGovern, at Biomolecular Archaeology Laboratory (www
.penn.museum/sites/biomoleculararchaeology/?page_id=247)
Handbook of Fermented Functional Foods, 2d ed., edited by Edward R.
Farnworth

Tempeh

"Time for Tempeh," by Phillip Rhodes, at *Cooking Light* (www
.cookinglight.com/food/vegetarian/time-for-tempeh
-00400000001121/)

Miso

Guide to Miso (http://miso.or.jp/misoonline/wp-content/uploads/2012
/09/miso-english-leaflet.pdf)

eight

The 21-Day Belly Fix: Days 11–21

SOLVE YOUR FOOD PUZZLE

Now that we've taken the top offenders out of your diet and replenished your gut with healthy bacteria, it's time to challenge your digestive tract. You're probably feeling less bloated and more comfortable in your abdominal region, as well as lighter overall. But let's be real—this is a rigid diet! Nobody wants to eat like this for the rest of his or her life, no matter how good he or she is feeling. It's time to begin solving the food puzzle.

This is the stage where we will begin to pinpoint your trigger foods— the ones you should eat infrequently, if at all. Since you're now eating a pretty wide variety of foods, there's a lot more flexibility from here on out. However, since you'll be adding in foods that are harder for many people to digest, pay close attention to how you feel as you add each ingredient. If any cause symptoms, eliminate them for at least six weeks and try again.

Here's how you'll eat for the next few days:

DAYS 11-13

Most of your routine will remain the same, however, beginning on day 11 you will reintroduce gluten-free grains.

Starting today, you can remove the kitchari from your diet. Instead, you'll begin including a half-cup of one of the following gluten-free grains or starchy vegetables: cooked brown rice, quinoa, oats, millet, wild rice, buckwheat, or white potatoes (including the skin). The carbohydrates in these foods will give you energy, while their fiber will help fill you up and sweep toxins from your digestive tract and minimize your body's post-meal insulin response, which decreases the production of inflammatory messengers in your body. What's more, gluten-free grains (in particular brown rice) in the diet have been linked with improved balance of gut bacteria.

You'll continue to avoid foods that contain wheat, barley, rye, and spelt. These grains contain gluten, a protein that is very difficult to digest and can even be seen by some people's bodies as a foreign invader. For most people, gluten is thought to be harmless—it makes dough elastic and helps give texture and shape to wheat products. For people with celiac disease, however, eating gluten rallies an immune response that in turn leads to a cascade of damage throughout the body. While only about 1 percent of the population has celiac disease, experts believe that far more people—as much as a third of the population—have some form of gluten sensitivity with symptoms ranging from gastrointestinal distress to migraines to skin disorders to foggy brain. This is a pattern I see in my practice. Clearly, many patients do not have celiac disease but are still gluten-intolerant. Gluten may also play a role in autoimmune diseases like type 1 diabetes and rheumatoid arthritis. Since there's no reliable test at this point to know for certain whether or not you are sensitive to gluten, I recommend eliminating it for the first few weeks of the plan to ensure that you're not unknowingly creating inflammation and any resulting distress.

Days 11–13 overview:

Meal/time	Food
Early morning (upon waking; 6:00–7:30 a.m.)	Diluted apple cider vinegar Warm ginger tea 1 brown rice cake with 1–2 teaspoons coconut oil and olive oil
Mid-morning (10:00 a.m.)	One protein shake (choose from one of the recipes in chapter 5 or create your own using 1 scoop protein powder and 1–2 servings produce); choose a shake that includes a banana or some wild blueberries for additional prebiotic fiber
Lunch (1:00 p.m.)	Green Juice Blend Coconut yogurt/kefir, tempeh, sauerkraut, kimchi, or kombucha
Dinner (5:00–6:00 p.m.)	Vegetables steamed or sautéed in olive oil or coconut oil (or you can use a miso-based sauce to help meet your probioitic requirement) 4–5 ounces white meat chicken or turkey, or white fish like flounder or sole **A half-cup gluten-free whole grains or starchy vegetable: brown rice, quinoa, oats, millet, polenta, grits, white potatoes with skin** Bone broth soup
Supplements	Glutamine powder (500 mg, once per day between meals); aloe vera juice (1–2 ounces, once per day); digestive enzymes (at least once per day with your heaviest meal or any other meal you need help with); one probiotic supplement (at least 500 cfu); 500 mg prebiotic powder added to mid-morning smoothie

CALORIES: ABOUT 1,600

DAYS 14–16

Red meat can be a trigger food for some people. Since it's generally higher in slower-to-digest fat than white meat like turkey and chicken, it is more likely to lead to symptoms such as indigestion, constipation, and gastrointestinal distress.

If you can tolerate red meat, great news: Eating it in moderation will provide you with enough protein to ditch the protein shakes. It's also an excellent source of vitamin B_6, vitamin B_{12}, selenium, zinc, and niacin and a good source of important minerals like iron. By keeping it to no more than four ounces one to two times per week, you can keep the heart health risks of eating too much red meat to a minimum.

On day 14, you'll eliminate the daily protein shake. Instead, you'll add a three-ounce serving of a lean cut of red meat like top sirloin, eye of round roast or steak, bottom round roast or steak, top round roast or steak, or sirloin tip side steaks to your lunch, pairing it with a serving of produce. On days 15 and 16, continue replacing the protein shake with a serving of lean red meat at lunch. Of course, if you don't like red meat or choose not to eat it for other reasons, you can skip this step altogether and replace your protein shake with a different lean protein, like fish or chicken (or continue with the protein shake if you're enjoying it).

For this trial—and as you continue to eat beef—I do recommend buying organic and grassfed beef. Cattle used for organic beef are raised without the use of growth hormones or pesticides, are fed only organic feed and grasses, and have unrestricted access to the outdoors. Grassfed beef is leaner and therefore lower in fat and calories than conventionally raised beef. It has higher levels of heart-healthy omega-3 fatty acids and is a good source of conjugated linoleic acid, a type of fat that may play a role in reducing cancer risk and insulin resistance, decreasing inflammation, and more.

Keep in mind that in other countries, beef is not the only source of red meat. My grandfather was a goat wholesaler in India. Goat is the preferred source of red meat in many other countries, and research is showing that goat meat is leaner, higher in iron and B vitamins, and easier to digest than beef. Other sources of red meat you may want to try include buffalo and venison.

At this stage you'll also move the green drink from lunchtime to the mid-morning, in place of the protein shake that you'll now be replacing with these other protein sources.

Beginning today, you'll also have a bit more freedom to find the right spot in your day for one serving of both prebiotic and probiotic foods— training wheels for when you'll be deciding what to eat for yourself at each meal, which starts in just a week. In addition, you'll begin to mix your prebiotic powder with water, since we've eliminated the protein drink you were blending it into up until now.

Days 14–16 overview:

Meal/time	Food
Early morning (upon waking; 6:00-7:30 a.m.)	Diluted apple cider vinegar Warm ginger tea 1 rice cake spread with 1–2 teaspoons coconut oil and olive oil
Mid morning (around 10:00 a.m.)	Green Juice Blend
Lunch (1:00 p.m.)	**3 ounces lean red meat** **1 serving fruit or vegetables**
Dinner (5:00–6:00 p.m.)	Vegetables steamed or sautéed in olive oil or coconut oil 4-5 ounces white meat chicken or turkey, or white fish like flounder or sole A half-cup gluten-free whole grains or starchy vegetable: brown rice, quinoa, oats, millet, polenta, grits, white potatoes with skin Bone broth soup
At some point during the day	One serving of probioitic foods: Coconut milk yogurt/kefir, sauerkraut, tempeh, miso, kimchi, or kombucha One serving of prebioitic foods: Bananas, wild blueberries, chicory root, Jerusalem artichokes, onion, or garlic
Supplements	Glutamine powder (500 mg, once per day between meals); aloe vera juice (1–2 ounces, once per day); digestive enzymes (at least once per day with your heaviest meal or any other meal you need help with); one probiotic supplement (at least 500 cfu); one scoop prebiotic powder **mixed with water**

CALORIES: ABOUT 1,600

DAYS 17-18

If you have a dairy allergy, you're probably well aware of it. An allergy is characterized by a range of immune system responses that can include anything from a rash to hives to wheezing and loss of consciousness; allergies can be life threatening. A dairy intolerance, however, is something that could easily have gone unnoticed up until now. Research shows that more than half the world's population has trouble breaking down lactose, the main carbohydrate found in milk. In my practice, dairy intolerance might cause nasal allergies in one patient and eczema in another. Dairy is a frequent cause of constipation as well as the first food eliminated in Ayurvedic and Chinese medicine when resting the gut. A person with lactose intolerance may experience more benign symptoms like nausea, gas, and bloating. Others are sensitive to casein, a protein in dairy foods, which can result in symptoms ranging from constipation, runny nose, and skin rashes to joint pain.

Beginning on day 17, you'll add one serving of dairy. I suggest eating it at mid-morning. Start with one cup of plain yogurt, since it's easier to digest than other dairy foods; if you tolerate that well, you can move on to other sources of dairy during the next few days. On day 18, you can include one cup of milk or one ounce of cheese. If you notice any symptoms, eliminate dairy again for six weeks. Once you feel that you can comfortably digest dairy, you should still limit your total dairy to one serving per day.

Today is also a good day to cut back on your oil calories. Since you're increasing fat and calories via the dairy, as just discussed, I suggest keeping the oil to one teaspoon maximum at each meal to account for the fat and calories added.

Overview of days 17–18:

Meal/time	Food
Early morning (upon waking; 6:00–7:30 a.m.)	Diluted apple cider vinegar Warm ginger tea 1 rice cake spread with 1 teaspoon total coconut oil and olive oil
Mid-morning (10:00 a.m.)	**One serving of dairy**
Lunch (1:00 p.m.)	Green Juice Blend One serving fruit or vegetables One serving red meat, chicken, turkey, or white fish

Dinner (5:00–6:00 p.m.)	Vegetables steamed or sautéed in olive oil or coconut oil 4–5 ounces white meat chicken or turkey, or white fish like flounder or sole A half-cup gluten-free whole grains or starchy vegetable: brown rice, quinoa, oats, millet, polenta, grits, or white potatoes with skin Bone broth soup
Supplements	Glutamine powder (500 mg, once per day between meals); aloe vera juice (1–2 ounces, once per day); digestive enzymes (at least once per day with your heaviest meal or any other meal you need help with); one probiotic supplement (at least 500 cfu); 500 mg prebiotic powder mixed with water

CALORIES: ABOUT 1,600

DAYS 19–21

In these last three days of the plan, you'll add in gluten. As we discussed earlier, gluten is a protein that is very difficult to digest and is even regarded by some people's bodies as a foreign invader. When you reintroduce gluten, you may experience symptoms ranging from gas and bloating to skin rashes, joint aches, fatigue, and brain fog. Continue to be mindful of any changes your body experiences.

I suggest swapping your morning rice cake spread with coconut oil and olive oil for a slice of whole-wheat bread. By consuming gluten first thing in the morning, you'll have the rest of the day to notice if anything seems off. Gluten intolerance symptoms can develop instantly or within a few hours, if not days. If after eating the bread you feel differently than you've felt over the past nine days, switch back to the rice cake and try bread (or another food with gluten in it like pasta) again in six weeks.

Once you've confirmed that you're okay with eating gluten, feel free to choose other gluten-containing foods as your half-cup of whole grains per day. Good choices include 1 or 2 slices of whole-wheat bread, 1 or 2 slices of spelt bread, a half-cup of barley, and a half-cup of whole-wheat pasta.

Again, even if you do not notice any changes with reintroducing gluten, limit your total gluten to one serving per day.

Days 19–21 overview:

Meal/time	Food
Early morning (upon waking; 6:00–7:30 a.m.)	Diluted apple cider vinegar Warm ginger tea 1 **slice of whole-wheat bread** with 1 teaspoon total coconut oil and olive oil
Mid-morning (10:00 a.m.)	One serving of dairy
Lunch (1:00 p.m.)	Green Juice Blend One serving of fruit or vegetables 3 ounces red meat, 4–5 ounces white meat or fish
Dinner (5:00–6:00 p.m.)	Vegetables steamed or sautéed in olive oil or coconut oil 4–5 ounces white meat chicken or turkey, or white fish like flounder or sole A half-cup gluten-free whole grains or starchy vegetable: brown rice, quinoa, oats, millet, polenta, grits, or white potatoes with skin Bone broth soup
Supplements	Glutamine powder (500 mg, once per day between meals); aloe vera juice (1–2 ounces, once per day); digestive enzymes (at least once per day with your heaviest meal or any other meal you need help with); one probiotic supplement (at least 500 cfu); 500 mg prebiotic powder mixed with water.

CALORIES: ABOUT 1,600

DAY 22 AND BEYOND

From day 22 on you can create your own mix of the foods (or follow my suggested menus). Here's how your diet should look:

- At least 1 serving of Green Juice Blend per day
- 1 fruit or vegetable at every meal (don't have fruit more than twice a day)
- 1 serving (½ cup to 1 cup) of whole grains per day

Introducing New Foods

I know you don't want to eat the same foods day in and day out. So what about those ingredients that I haven't included, like eggs, peanut butter, and tofu? Just because they haven't been in the plan up until now doesn't mean they're off-limits. Once you've gotten comfortable with the regimen and have a good understanding of your trigger foods, it's totally fine to experiment with other ingredients. Simply swap in the food you'd like to try where it seems most fitting—eggs in place of meat, for instance—and include it in your diet for two to three consecutive days. Carefully track any symptoms that may appear; if there are none, you can include the food in your regular rotation.

- 2 servings of lean protein (chicken, turkey, fish, lean red meat, or eggs) per day
- 1 serving of dairy per day
- At least 1 fermented food per day
- At least 2 servings of healthy fat (avocado, olives, nuts, olive oil, coconut oil, avocado oil, or peanut oil) per day
- Continue with the supplement regimen

The beauty of the 21-Day Belly Fix is that the mix of foods provided keep your total sugar low and minimize your exposure to gluten and dairy while adding lots of great probiotics and prebiotics and rebuilding your gut lining. By following this plan, you should be healthy for years to come, not just 21 days.

SAMPLE MENUS

Sample Day 1

Early Morning

Diluted apple cider vinegar

Warm ginger tea

1 slice of whole-wheat bread with 1 teaspoon coconut oil and olive oil

Mid-Morning:

1 single-serving container of Greek yogurt

½ cup blueberries

Lunch:

Green Juice Blend

3 cups sautéed baby arugula and ¼ cup sliced red onion topped with ¼ avocado, 3 ounces grilled chicken and miso dressing

Dinner:

Red and green pepper slices sautéed in canola oil with 3 ounces lean beef with ½ cup brown rice

Bone broth soup

Supplements

Glutamine powder (500 mg, once per day between meals); aloe vera juice (1–2 ounces, once per day); digestive enzymes (at least once per day with your heaviest meal or any other meal you need help with); one probiotic supplement (at least 500 cfu); one scoop prebiotic powder.

Sample Day 2

Early Morning

Diluted apple cider vinegar

Warm ginger tea

1 slice of whole-wheat bread with 1 teaspoon coconut oil and olive oil

Mid-Morning

1 cup plain kefir blended with 1 medium banana

Lunch

    Green Juice Blend

    Tempeh Reuben (see page 215)

Dinner

    ½ butternut squash baked and stuffed with ½ cup quinoa mixed with ½ cup sautéed baby spinach and 1 broiled fillet of sole with a squeeze of lemon

    Bone broth soup

Supplements

    Glutamine powder (500 mg, once per day between meals); aloe vera juice (1–2 ounces, once per day); digestive enzymes (at least once per day with your heaviest meal or any other meal you need help with); one probiotic supplement (at least 500 cfu); 500 mg prebiotic powder.

Sample Day 3

Early Morning

    Diluted apple cider vinegar

    Warm ginger tea

    1 slice of whole-wheat bread with 1 teaspoon coconut oil and olive oil

Mid-Morning

    1 container of coconut milk yogurt with ½ cup sliced strawberries

Lunch

    Green Juice Blend

    1 large egg scrambled in vegetable oil with 2 cups baby spinach, ½ cup sliced white button mushrooms topped with ¼ avocado

    1 slice whole-wheat toast

Dinner

Greek vegetables and chicken: ⅓ cup chopped green pepper, ⅓ cup chopped red onion, ⅓ cup chopped tomato sautéed, topped with grilled 4-ounce chicken breast and 1 ounce crumbled feta cheese

Bone broth soup

Supplements

Glutamine powder (500 mg, once per day between meals); aloe vera juice (1–2 ounces, once per day); digestive enzymes (at least once per day with your heaviest meal or any other meal you need help with); one probiotic supplement (at least 500 cfu); 500 mg prebiotic powder.

SHOPPING LIST

Gluten-free grains: brown rice, quinoa, oats, millet, buckwheat

Organic grassfed beef

Dairy: milk, plain yogurt, cheese

Gluten-containing grains: whole-wheat bread, whole-wheat pasta, barley

nine

The 21-Day Belly Fix— for Good

Now that you've completed the 21-Day Belly Fix, I want to give you the tools to help you customize the plan to your body's own special needs. When patients come into my office, it often takes no more than a normal consultation and possibly a few tests to help determine what dietary tweaks will be the most helpful for them. Since I can't see your physical symptoms or hear about your experiences, it's hard—no, impossible—for me to diagnose you in any way. However, I have created an assessment tool to help you narrow down what, if any, alterations you should make to the 21-Day Belly Fix plan to help you reach optimal gut health. Once you take the quiz below, you'll tally up the answers and follow the guide at the end of the chapter to tailor the plan just for you.

Please keep in mind that this tool does not take the place of a consultation with a doctor who can run tests and use his or her years of experience and schooling to make an educated diagnosis. Rather, it can help you narrow down a cause of your discomfort and give you some suggestions as to what changes might benefit you. I do recommend that you discuss your findings with a qualified medical professional before you make any long-term changes in your diet.

THE DR. TAZ 21-DAY BELLY FIX TEST

Take a look at the test below. Give yourself one point for every yes answer and zero points for every no. Remember, you should take this test after you finish the 21-Day Belly Fix.

1. Do you crave carbohydrates like bread, sugar, and fruit? Y   N
2. Do you have itching in your rectal area? Y   N
3. Do you have recurring skin or nail fungal infections like athlete's foot, vaginal infections, jock itch, or ringworm? Y   N
4. Do you have frequent bloating or gas? Y   N
5. Do you regularly deal with diarrhea or constipation? Y   N
6. Do you have itching, flaking in your scalp? Y   N
7. Do you suffer from rosacea or psoriasis? Y   N
8. Do you feel bloating, cramps in the lower abdomen, or other symptoms within 2 hours of eating milk products? Y   N
9. Do you struggle with constipation only? Y   N
10. Have you been diagnosed with IBS? Y   N
11. Are you of Asian, African, Arab, Jewish, Greek, or Italian descent? Y   N
12. Do you struggle with joint aches and pains? Y   N
13. Have you been diagnosed with an autoimmune disorder like type 1 diabetes or rheumatoid arthritis? Y   N
14. Do you have diarrhea or loose stools more than three times per week? Y   N
15. Do you have brain fog? Y   N
16. Do you have fatigue? Y   N
17. Do you have issues with focus, anxiety, or depression? Y   N
18. Do you have reflux or heartburn? Y   N
19. Did you feel better off without meat? Y   N
20. Are you experiencing hair loss? Y   N

Score on 1–6:
Score on 6–12:

Score on 10–17:
Score on 18–19:
Total score:

As you answer these questions, look back at your symptom diary to see where in the 21-Day Belly Fix plan you felt better. For example, did you notice an improvement in your reflux or heartburn as you took dairy away—and a return when it was reintroduced? Did your constipation clear when you weren't eating meat but return when you added it back in?

Let's look at your score, section by section. Each answer provides clues on how to modify the 21-Day Belly Fix plan going forward.

First, review your answers to questions 1–6. If you scored 6 points here, there's a good chance you have a gut microbiology condition called **candida.** If you scored 4 or 5 points on questions 1–6, candida is still a possibility. Candida is an overgrowth or an abundance of yeast in the gut. Yeast is usually found in small amounts in your body, and your immune system is usually pretty good at keeping it in check. However, chronic antibiotic use, prescription medications, and sugary diets all can throw off your body's balance and contribute to an increase in the body's candida population, which can cause many of the symptoms and diagnosis in questions 1–6. While there are many candida diets out there, I often find them very hard to follow and often too restrictive. Instead, I work with my patients to help lower the candida load without eliminating an unnecessary amount of ingredients from their diets. Here are the alterations you can make to help the 21-Day Belly Fix work for you if you have candida:

- Limit fruit to one serving per day; avoiding all refined sugars and carbohydrates as well. The reason? Sugar provides fuel for yeast; having it in your body in excess will make it easier for the yeast to multiply. When choosing carbohydrate-rich foods, be extra careful to select unprocessed ones like rolled oats, buckwheat, brown rice, and quinoa.

- Restrict dairy to no more than three servings per week. Dairy will often trigger a candida overgrowth.
- Keep consumption of fermented food to no more than three times per week. Some experts believe that excess consumption of fermented foods can also lead to candida overgrowth.
- Season your food with the following flavorings, all proven to have antifungal properties: raw garlic, cloves, cinnamon, thyme, and lemon juice. See page 217 for a Greek-inspired dressing made of candida-preventing ingredients that works well on vegetables, meat, and fish.

I also use many herbal supplement remedies for candida, including garlic, oregano oil, berberine, or pau d'arco. Each of these have side effects, so they should be discussed with your doctor before beginning.

If your score on questions 6–12 falls between 4 and 6, you may benefit from decreasing or eliminating your intake of **dairy.** Dairy is a predominant protein in our standard American diet, with children in particular overconsuming in the form of ice cream, macaroni and cheese, and other milk products. As adults, we are no different. My mom ran and still owns an ice cream store in Atlanta, and as teenagers, my sisters and I would sneak tastes of ice cream whenever we could. It is no surprise to me that once I left home, my limited access to dairy allowed me to lose weight and get rid of my acne. I am almost fifteen pounds lighter in my forties than I was as a teenager. I still love ice cream—but it is now the occasional treat.

The 21-Day Belly Fix includes a once-daily dose of dairy, which you began on day 17. If you scored between 4 and 6 on questions 6–12, shift to using a lactose-free (or low-lactose) option for one week. If even the low-lactose dairy options are giving you a problem, it may be other compounds in the dairy, like the milk proteins casein or whey, that are bothersome. You'll then go on to remove dairy completely, replacing your daily serving with a coconut-based non-dairy milk product. Here's how you'll proceed:

First, test out low-lactose dairy for one week. Good options: lactose-free yogurt from Green Valley, Horizon Organic lactose-free milk,

or Cabot cheddar. In addition, any cheese with zero grams of carbohydrates listed is extremely low in lactose; any yogurt that contains "live and active cultures" is already partially broken down by
enzymes and is likely to be tolerated in moderation.

If after a week you're still having trouble tolerating your daily serving
of dairy, eliminate it completely, replacing your daily serving with
coconut milk or cultured coconut milk (also known as yogurt).

The Dairy-Free Trap: The biggest challenge for my patients that are
dairy-free is the drop in protein, since many patients rely on dairy
as a main source of the nutrient. If you find that you are struggling
with alternative sources of protein, consider keeping your protein
shakes in the plan or fortify the alternative milks like rice, hemp,
coconut, or almond with additional protein (in the form of powder) at least once per day. Some non-dairy milks are now fortified
with protein; look for these products (one example is So Delicious
Almond Plus). Worried about the calcium in milk? People are
often surprised to hear that we can get plenty of calcium from leafy
greens, nuts, and fish that contain small bones (foods like broccoli,
kale, almonds, and sardines are all good sources). As insurance,
make sure that your alternative milk is fortified with calcium; look
for one with at least 25 percent of your daily need per serving.

Now take a look at your answers to questions 10–17. If you scored
between 5 and 7 points on this portion of the test, you may have an issue
tolerating **gluten.** As a result, a diet free of the protein found in wheat,
barley, spelt, and rye may be the answer for you. As we discussed in chapter 9, in some people, eating gluten triggers an immune response that can
cause symptoms ranging from severe intestinal damage and nutrient malabsorption to migraines and foggy brain. Please note that if you suspect
celiac disease, it is crucial you get tested for celiac right away—before you
eliminate gluten from your diet (without gluten in your system, your body
won't create antibodies to it—one of the very things that's used to diagnose celiac disease). If you've already ruled out celiac disease but notice a
marked improvement in symptoms when you remove gluten from your

diet, you may have non-celiac gluten sensitivity. To keep your symptoms in check, you may also benefit from adhering to a strictly gluten-free diet. Here's how to adjust the 21-Day Belly Fix accordingly:

1. Remove the whole-wheat bread you added on day 19, instead sticking with gluten-free grain foods like brown rice cakes, brown rice, quinoa, millet, buckwheat, polenta, and wild rice.

2. Be careful to avoid hidden sources of gluten. All of the following words on an ingredient label should raise a red flag: barley, bulgur, durum, farina, faro, kamut, malt, oats (non-certified gluten-free oats are almost always contaminated with gluten), rye, seitan, semolina, spelt, and wheat germ. It's also found in soy sauce, beer, cereals, and other places you might not expect it.

3. If you do accidentally get "glutened," there are digestive enzymes that help break down the gluten protein that you may want to keep on hand. These enzymes contain diphenylarsinic acid (DPAA) and can prevent the effects of gluten from sneaking into your diet.

4. Watch the Gluten-Free Trap: I always warn my patients that the biggest issue with many gluten-free diets is relying heavily on substitutes for bread, crackers, pretzels—in other words, "gluten-free junk." Since these substitutes are often loaded with sugar (not to mention calories), overdoing them can lead to candida, as we previously discussed.

If your overall score was 15–20, you may have a condition called **small intestinal bacterial overgrowth.** With SIBO, any of the symptoms on the Dr. Taz 21-Day Belly Fix Test are fair game—you may benefit from tweaking your diet to make sure it's low in FODMAPs (fermentable, oligo-, di-, mono-saccharides, and polyols)—this includes foods that contain a high level of the fruit sugar fructose as well as of the milk sugar lactose, among other food compounds, which are poorly digested and can trigger fermentation in the belly. The benefit of using the 21-Day Belly Fix rather than jumping headfirst into a low-FODMAP plan is that you've had the opportunity to allow your gut to heal and to identify some trigger foods that may be responsible for SIBO. But if IBS symptoms are still plaguing you and there's no real indication of what may be causing them, it may make sense for you to adjust your 21-Day Belly Fix by supplementing it with what we've learned works in the low-FODMAP plan. Here are the tweaks you'll make:

Choose low-lactose or lactose-free dairy like Green Valley yogurt, Horizon Organic lactose-free milk, or Cabot Cheddar cheese.

When choosing fruits (including drinks and smoothies including fruit) favor low-FODMAP choices like berries, bananas, cantaloupe, and citrus. Avoid stone fruit like peaches, plums, cherries, nectarines, and avocado as well as apples, pears, and dates.

Stick with gluten-free grains like brown rice, brown rice cakes, quinoa, polenta, and millet.

Avoid onions and garlic as well as broccoli, cauliflower, Brussels sprouts, beets, and cabbage. Low-FODMAP vegetables include cucumber, eggplant, winter squash, tomatoes, pumpkin, yams, leafy greens, carrots, and corn.

Continue to use fermented foods and bone broth soups to rebuild and rebalance intestinal flora.

For a thorough list of high- and low-FODMAPs foods, there are many resources available. Look online for the most up-to-date information; you can also download an app to help you out in the grocery store or at restaurants.

SIBO is one condition that may need treatment with antibiotics. If you continue to have symptoms even after the changes to your diet, please see your doctor for an evaluation.

Finally, look at your answers to questions 18 and 19. If you answered yes, you may need to become a vegetarian. Even if meat doesn't bother your belly, you just may be happiest adjusting the plan for a vegetarian palate. This is, of course, a choice rather than a diagnosis—but many people are opting for vegetarian diets nowadays, and I want to make sure the

21-Day Belly Fix is accessible to everyone who chooses it. However, even if you like the taste of meat, you may have trouble digesting it—red meat in particular—noticing with reintroduction of meat a return of joint pain, constipation, and reflux. Look back at your symptom diary to see if you noticed these symptoms return as we introduced meat into the 21-Day Belly Fix. If so, I suggest you make the following adjustments (I'll start at day 1, just in case you want to keep it vegetarian from the get-go):

Day 5: Instead of bone broth soup, use the miso broth recipe on page 218.

Day 6: Instead of adding lean meat, use a serving (around ⅓ cup) of lentils, chickpeas, or tempeh.

Day 14: Instead of adding red meat, add another serving of the plant-based proteins from above.

Day 17: If you're lacto vegetarian, meaning you eat dairy foods, you don't have to change anything. If you're vegan, meaning you eat no animal products including dairy, eggs, and honey, you'll add in an additional serving of coconut milk–based dairy replacement (milk, cultured milk/yogurt, or kefir) in place of the cow's milk dairy recommended at this point.

The Vegetarian Trap: I have not forgotten question 20; hair loss, after all, is part of what started my journey into integrative medicine. One of the biggest traps for vegetarians is the lack of protein in their diets, which can often trigger deficiencies in iron, B vitamins, and amino acids all most visibly necessary in hair growth and maintenance. As a vegetarian, make sure you are counting your protein grams and getting at least 50 grams of protein per day. You may also want to supplement you diet with the following:

B complex that includes 1,000 micrograms of B_{12}

Iron in the form of an iron chelate, 30 mg per day. You may have to experiment with different forms of iron to make sure that they do not cause constipation.

An additional protein shake or smoothie to help you get roughly 46–50 grams of protein per day (the average amounts women and men need, respectively). As well, make sure that you're choosing protein-rich foods in place of meat. Vegetarian protein sources include garbanzo beans, black beans, kidney beans, tempeh, eggs, peanuts, walnuts, almonds, cashews, ricotta cheese, cottage cheese, yogurt, and peas.

ten

Seven Stress Soothers
for a Happy Gut

A few years back, for an entire year, my husband greeted me each morning not with a kiss but with the most horrible retching. Some mornings, his nausea and abdominal pain led to vomiting. At the time, the pace of our lives was frantic. He was starting his practice. I was starting mine *and* working in the ER. Both of us were putting in fourteen-hour days and trying to be loving parents to our children, both of whom were under two.

He got tested for food allergies—none. Thinking he might be lactose-intolerant or gluten-sensitive, I put him on dairy- and gluten-free diets. No change. The natural remedies I brought home didn't help; neither did the medications I prescribed. I drove myself nuts trying to diagnose his symptoms. Was it reflux? Diverticulitis? A hiatal hernia?

After about six months of this, we went on vacation. In Cancun, for one lovely week, his symptoms vanished even as he enjoyed his "vacation diet" loaded with sugars, fat, and alcohol. *What?* His nausea, gone, on a steady diet of dessert and cocktails? Maybe he was sleeping better. I was just glad his ailment seemed to have cleared up.

When we returned to Atlanta, however, so did his symptoms. The very next morning, in fact.

But life went on. Pushing through the nausea and discomfort, my husband finally set up his practice. He worked less punishing hours, got enough sleep, ate healthy meals at home instead of fast food between patients, and started hitting the gym regularly again. And then, one morning, instead of his usual I'm-gonna-be-sick face, I was greeted with a kiss. His "mystery ailment" was gone.

In hindsight, there was no mystery: As his stress eased, his gut responded. I was familiar with the research that links stress to a variety of gut woes, from nausea and heartburn to flareups of serious inflammatory bowel diseases like Crohn's disease and ulcerative colitis as well as IBS. During that frantic period of our lives, however, neither of us had even considered that stress was literally making him sick to his stomach. But there's no doubt about it, because the symptoms return when his stress boils over.

My husband and I—both doctors—learned something from this episode. Your gut needs more than a good diet, regular exercise, and the right nutritional supplements. It needs peace. And the key to peace is creating, and sticking to, a stress-management plan. It adds pleasure to your life, takes fifteen minutes a day max, and is something you can use to begin healing your stress—and gut—today. This chapter shows you how.

STRESS BEGINS IN THE BODY

Many people believe that stress is caused by personal circumstances. After all, our times of biggest stress coincide with major life changes that trigger *acute* stress, such as death, job loss, and breakups, or the *routine* stress of continuing challenges—job, bills, kids, a long commute, caring for aging parents.

To researchers who study stress, however, its root is not in our circumstances, however challenging. It's in our bodies. To such experts, stress is the body's automatic physiologic reaction to circumstances.

Faced with a threat to your survival—say, a car hurtling toward you from the opposite lane of the highway—your body goes into caveman mode. Automatically, instantaneously, cells in the nervous and endocrine systems act in concert to prepare the body to fight or flee. This cascade of hormonal changes and physiological responses is called the *stress response*. Your pupils dilate, the better to see the threat. Your heart and respiration rates accelerate. Blood flow to your skeletal muscles increases, so you can fight or run.

We need this hard-wired response to danger to react quickly when our lives are at stake. However, the stress response is often tripped by false alarms. The part of the brain the initiates the automatic part of the stress response, called the amygdala, can't distinguish a real threat to survival— say, that oncoming car—from a *perceived* threat. Mistaking the two can keep the stress response "switched on" for weeks, months, or even years. Your body never has a chance to return to a state of rest, which is harmful to your physical and emotional well-being.

Integrative medicine views stress not just as life challenges and their management but also as a chemical process that leads to disease. Fatigue, illness, and surgery are *physical stressors* that tax the body; life-based or *psychosocial stressors,* large or small, temporary or long-term, wear us down mentally, emotionally, and spiritually. *Metabolic stressors* tax our body systems. These include chronic inflammation, hormonal imbalance, exposure to toxins, and too few or too many calories. The damage—either direct or indirect—involves every system in the body and includes a spike in the stress hormone cortisol, reduced blood flow to vital organs like the stomach and liver, and the depletion of vital nutrients such as B vitamins and amino acids.

THIS IS YOUR GUT ON STRESS

When stress is strong enough to trigger the fight-or-flight response, your belly is in for trouble. Digestion slows or even stops so that your body can devote its full resources to the perceived threat. Stress hormones can also stimulate intestinal muscles, leading to cramping and diarrhea, or slow them down, leading to constipation.

In other words, eating and stress don't mix. If you gobble breakfast in your car during your long commute to work or have lunch at your desk as you stress about your relationship, your presentation, or simply how you'll get everything done today, your gut is receiving an unhealthy message: THREAT AHEAD. STOP DIGESTING. If you think about it, this makes sense. We normally don't eat and fight (or flee) at the same time.

Slowed or stopped digestion can cause heartburn, nausea, or other gut symptoms. And even if you're eating a healthy meal, since your digestive system isn't functioning at its peak, it won't absorb all the nutrients in your food.

Eating in response to stress can make things worse. When a digestive system slowed by stress must break down large amounts of food, the typical result is serious digestive discomfort ranging from heartburn to gas.

Stress can also change the permeability of the intestine, which gives undigested food particles and bacteria access to immune cells. The resulting inflammation can cause serious inflammatory bowel disorders in people predisposed to them.

Although stress does not cause IBD, it can aggravate the symptoms of the disease and may be a key cause of flareups. In fact, stress and major negative life events were more likely to cause flares than physical factors like infections or nonsteroidal anti-inflammatory drugs (NSAIDs) such as aspirin and ibuprofen, according to a 2010 study published in *The American Journal of Gastroenterology*. Peptic ulcers aren't caused by stress either—the culprit is *H. pylori* bacteria or the use of NSAIDs. But just as with IBD, research has found that stress may predispose a person with *H. pylori* to ulcers.

Chronic stress may even contribute to an imbalance of gut bacteria. In a 2011 study in mice published in *Brain, Behavior, and Immunity,* researchers at Ohio State University examined the effects of stress-induced changes to the gut microbiome on health. Mice that shared a cage with aggressive mice were found to exhibit a reduction of beneficial gut bacteria, an overgrowth of harmful gut bacteria, and a reduced diversity of the gut microbiome overall. This caused gut inflammation in the timid mice and increased their vulnerability to infection.

TRY A "STRESS JAM" TO SHORT-CIRCUIT THE STRESS RESPONSE

While you can't control stressful events, you *can* change your perception of them, which in turn changes how you react to them. This reframing can short-circuit the body's stress response. A key strategy in such "stress-jamming" is to learn to elicit the opposite of the stress response: the *relaxation response*.

Dr. Herbert Benson, director emeritus of the Benson-Henry Institute for Mind Body Medicine at Massachusetts General Hospital, coined this term almost forty years ago. Induced by such simple techniques as deep breathing, meditation, and repetitive prayer, the relaxation response is a state of deep physiologic rest. Decades of research has shown that it can slow the breathing rate, relax the muscles, and reduce blood pressure, thereby helping to counteract the toxic effects of chronic stress. Fortunately, you can trigger the relaxation response by using techniques like those mentioned above.

Like a successful exercise plan, a successful stress-management plan is one you like and use. There are so many pleasurable stress-management techniques that you're bound to have (or discover) a favorite or three.

In my view, a good stress-management plan has two tiers—a daily plan of 15–20 minutes to ease the stresses of everyday life and a weekly routine that might include a massage, a yoga class or acupuncture session (see page 152), a get-together with friends, or alone time to relax and recharge.

Many of the techniques below have been found to elicit the relaxation response. Any would fit nicely into your custom-designed plan. Most take less than five minutes and can be done anytime, anywhere—at home, at work, even sitting in traffic or on public transportation. Read through the list, then pick one or two that you'll commit to each day and at least one you'll use once a week.

Deep Breathing

The 1:4:7 Breath

The next time you're stressed, tune in to your breathing. Most likely, your breaths will be short and shallow, and your shoulders may rise and fall with each breath. Or your chest may feel tight or compressed, making it hard to draw a full breath.

Consciously slowing your breathing is a time-honored stress-jamming tactic. Yogis in India have known this for thousands of years, using *pranayama*—translated as, "control of the life force"—to benefit their physical and spiritual well-being.

The 1:4:7 breath is an adaptation of a breathing technique found in ancient Sanskrit texts. It's so simple and effective that I use it to re-center nearly every day. Within just a cycle or two, blood flow to the gut increases and blood pressure and cortisol levels fall. This technique also improves production of digestive enzymes and improves neurotransmitter balance, including gut-relaxing serotonin.

- Sit on the floor Indian-style or in a chair with your hands on your lap.
- Close your eyes and place your tongue behind your bottom teeth.
- With your mouth closed, inhale deeply and slowly through your nose, blowing your belly out. Hold that breath to a silent count of 4.
- Exhale slowly through your open mouth, flattening your belly down to your navel. Hold for a silent count of 7.
- Repeat the inhale/exhale cycle for a total of 4 cycles.

Meditation

Mindfulness Meditation

I treat a lot of high-powered, stressed-out, Type-A patients. And at some point, most tell me, flat out, that meditation just isn't for them. Knowing that they were picturing incense and lotus positions, I'd ask, gently, if they wanted a more peaceful life or at least a pain-free belly. At that point, most

How I Manage Stress

I have a high tolerance for stress. But I also have a lot on my plate, and it's all too easy for my life to become unbalanced by it. I've long since recognized my personal warning signs of stress: heart palpitations, sleepless nights, obsessive worry about situations I can't control. Oh, and compulsive list-making. My lists are on paper, and I make separate lists for home, kids, office, and deadlines. As the lists get longer, I know it is time to pull back.

Because my days are so demanding, I've found that early morning is the best time for me to practice my daily stress management. I love getting up before everyone else to journal, pray, and read uplifting books. (Two of my favorites are *Every Day a Friday* by Joel Osteen and *The Happiness Project* by Gretchen Rubin.)

Exercise is part of my early-morning routine, too. If I don't work out before my day officially begins, I may get too busy to fit it in, and that would be a disaster. Without regular exercise, stress affects me more quickly and intensely.

Throughout the day, I rely on the 1:4:7 breath to re-center. And at night, when the kids are in bed and I have a few precious minutes of "me" time, I decompress with journaling, prayer, or deep breathing.

My weekly stress-management routine includes massage and acupuncture. I *love* acupuncture—in fact, I perform it on myself! I think acupuncture appeals to me because my job is very mental—I'm constantly "in my head," thinking, calculating, processing. Using acupuncture to unblock the gallbladder, liver, and kidney meridians, which are associated with stress, offers instant tranquillity, helping me regain my balance and focus. I place about thirty needles throughout my forehead and face, leave them there for about twenty-five minutes while I catch a quick nap, toss them in the trash (they're disposable!), and carry on, relaxed, refreshed, and recharged.

grudgingly tried the simple meditation technique below—and got hooked.

If you're a skeptic, bypass the more "out there" transcendental and zen forms and opt for mindfulness meditation, popularized by Dr. Jon Kabat-Zinn in the 1990s. This simple, practical technique is my personal favorite because you can do it anywhere and no one ever has to know.

Mindfulness meditation is the practice of becoming aware of and staying in the present moment. Just ten minutes can help ease your mind—and belly. In a study of seventy-five women with IBS published in *The American Journal of Gastroenterology,* researchers at the University of North Carolina School of Medicine in Chapel Hill divided the women into two groups. One group received training in mindfulness-based stress reduction. The other was assigned to an IBS support group. Both groups attended weekly sessions plus a half-day retreat.

After eight weeks, both groups reported that their IBS symptoms were less severe. But the mindful meditation group's improvement was truly dramatic—a 26.4 percent reduction in severity, compared to 6.2 percent for the control group. Three months after the study, the mindfulness group's improvement actually increased—a 38.2 percent reduction in symptoms, compared to 11.8 percent for the control group.

Below is a basic mindfulness meditation. Here's how to do it.

1. Sit in a chair with your spine erect. Keep your feet flat on the floor and shoulder-width apart.

2. Close your eyes and breathe naturally. After a few breaths, try breathing with your abdomen only. Slowly, your breath will deepen as you practice.

3. Begin to quiet your mind. It's natural for your stressed-out mind to "chatter." Don't fight it. Now, begin to imagine your thoughts as cars on a highway, speeding by quickly. As a thought enters your mind, let it pass quickly—don't dwell on it. Continue watching your thoughts speed by, letting them come and go. Continue to bring your mind back to your breath.

5. Begin with 5 minutes, progressing at your own pace to 10–15 minutes.

You can't do this on your daily commute if you drive to work, of course. But you can do a driving meditation, in which you use your time in the car to clear your mind. A driving meditation is especially helpful if you tend to choke down an unhealthy grab-and-go meal in your car, text and check your e-mail at traffic lights, and station-surf while you drive. You can do a driving meditation in silence or pop in a CD of meditation music. Keep your eyes on the road, but focus on your breathing, gently turning away obtrusive thoughts or worries.

To take your meditation practice with you, download meditation audiobooks or apps to your smartphone or iPad. Some of my favorites include *Meditation without Borders* (iTunes) and *Guided Mindfulness Meditation, Series 1* by Jon Kabat-Zinn (Sounds True).

Aromatherapy

Follow Your Nose to Tranquillity

With a busy practice, a lively family, and a full plate of public appearances, you bet I experience stress. Boarding a red-eye flight after a full day of treating patients, staying up all night with a sick child, or treating a patient with a challenging ailment can cause stress-induced headaches or abdominal pain.

Aromatherapy—the therapeutic use of essential oils for healing—is the quickest and most pleasurable tool in my stress-management kit. Within a minute of massaging a drop of peppermint essential oil into my temples for headaches or a drop of lavender or sandalwood onto my abdomen for abdominal pain, my serenity returns.

People all over the world have inhaled the essential oils of certain plants or massaged them into their skin for thousands of years, from China and India to ancient Greece and Rome. Modern science still hasn't unlocked aromatherapy's healing powers. It may be that smell receptors in the nose communicate with certain regions in the brain that store emotions and memories. Inhaling the molecules of essential oils may stimulate these brain regions (called the amygdala and the hippocampus) for a positive effect on physical and emotional well-being. Other research speculates that the molecules in these oils may interact in the blood with hormones or enzymes.

Recent studies continue to reveal fascinating findings about the link between our sense of smell and our moods. For example, a 2013 study published in *The Journal of Neuroscience* found that people with anxiety can experience a heightened sense of smell. That's okay. You can use your anxiety-sharpened sense of smell to ease bothersome side effects of stress, including indigestion.

Pick up a bottle or two of essential oils from your local natural-foods store. When stress strikes, uncap and take a whiff. I recommend sandalwood and lavender oils to relax your gut and improve digestion and peppermint oil to ease stress-induced headaches. Or try the aromatherapy inhalers found in health food stores. These look like those mentholated inhalers people use for nasal congestion. Some inhalers are "blank," so you can fill them with your favorite oils; others come pre-filled with essential oils. I use the inhalers—they're quick and convenient.

Acupressure

Press Away Stress

If you're in the first trimester of pregnancy and battling nausea, take it from me—acupressure works. My first pregnancy was memorable for the horrible nausea I endured the first month or two. Nothing helped (not even ginger tea!) until I placed acupressure bands on acupuncture point pericardium 6, or PC6. Located slightly below the inner wrist, PC6 is a key point for regulating nausea. The bands provided almost instant relief and helped me make it through those tough months of early pregnancy.

Acupressure works much like acupuncture. According to practitioners of traditional Chinese medicine, this ancient technique improves physical and emotional well-being by balancing qi, the life energy that runs along twelve meridians in the body. Each meridian begins at the fingertips, then ties in with the brain to specific organs or organ systems. Illness results when meridians are blocked or out of balance. Acupressure, much like acupuncture, restores that balance.

Acupuncture Relieves a Raging Gut

Newly diagnosed with Crohn's disease, my patient was clear: He did not want to change his diet, was too busy to exercise, and had no interest in swallowing the supplements I wanted to prescribe. To my surprise, he *did* agree to three months of acupuncture sessions, once or twice a week.

Unlike some of my patients, he had no problem with my inserting needles at the digestive points on his abdomen, arms, and legs. In fact, he looked forward to his sessions as an opportunity to unwind and recharge. And after just ninety days, he was flare-free, with no recurrence of his disease.

In study after study, acupuncture has been found to improve symptoms of some inflammatory bowel disorders, including ulcerative colitis, Crohn's disease, gastritis, and reflux. In a 2007 study, researchers at the University of Arizona divided thirty people with reflux who still had symptoms while taking a potent prescription acid-blocking medication into two groups. The first group got the medication twice daily. The other group received the drug once a day and also received acupuncture—three times a week for the first two weeks, then twice a week for the rest of the four-week study.

Compared to the group that received the double dose of the drug, those in the acupuncture group reported that their daytime heartburn, nighttime heartburn, and acid regurgitation improved significantly—and after only ten sessions. While the mechanism by which acupuncture helped isn't yet clear, researchers speculated that it may reduce stomach acid and speed up digestion so that less acid backs up into the esophagus.

If your digestive symptoms include heartburn, cramping, abdominal pain, or nausea, acupuncture may provide relief, especially if your gut diary shows that stress precipitates your symptoms. Choose a licensed acupuncturist—such professionals have "L. Ac." after their names. That means they attended a four-year acupuncture school and are licensed by the state. Commit to at least three sessions before you decide whether acupuncture is improving your symptoms.

While there are hundreds of acupressure points on the body, three are commonly used by practitioners of traditional Chinese medicine. As I mentioned, PC6 is located on your inner wrist, on the same side as the palm. Large intestine 4 (L14) is located in the fleshy web between your thumb and forefinger. Spleen 6 (SP6) lies slightly above your inner ankle-bone in the lower calf muscle.

If you're plagued by digestive issues such as nausea, heartburn, or constipation, this simple acupressure technique can provide temporary relief.

1. Locate each acupressure point, using the pictures to guide you.
2. Using the index finger and thumb of your opposing hand, apply steady, firm, direct pressure to any of these three points for five minutes. You can also place a small magnet or seed, perhaps from an apple, on the point and use tape to keep it in place.

Prayer

Release and Find Peace

In ancient times, the healers of a community were the priests and religious elders. The connection between feeling close to a higher power and being healthy has long been debated and indirectly proven. If you are plagued by chronic mental stress, prayer is a way to release negative emotions, reclaim your connection to the universe, and find healing.

Research shows a correlation between people who pray and lower stress levels. Dr. Benson has said that regular prayer, along with general stress management, can reduce visits to doctors and other health professionals by 50 percent. How might praying relieve stress? People who pray are typically connected to a religious community, and that community provides social support, which research has identified as a vital ingredient of physical and emotional well-being. Regular churchgoers not only receive support from their community; they give it, and altruism has also been found to have beneficial effects on health and happiness.

Prayer is very personal. There's no "right" way to pray, and no specific prayer you need to use. No matter how you engage in it, simply taking the action can provide shelter from the storm of stress.

Yoga

The Pose That Refreshes

In 2002, in the midst of a stressful residency and then an equally stressful ER job, I took my first yoga class and discovered true peace and joy. So much so that somehow, in spite of my impossible schedule, I received training to become a certified yoga instructor. Life would only get crazier, I reasoned. Later in my career, I might not be able to fit in a regular yoga class, so I'd better teach myself.

I'm so glad I did. Having kids and a busy practice does make it hard to get to a yoga studio, so I do my *vinyasa* yoga workout at home at least once a week. Someday, I plan to practice yoga daily. But for now, even once a week clears my mind, lowers my stress, and melts away any lingering back and neck aches after a hectic day.

A growing body of scientific research that concludes that the practice offers relief from a variety of health ailments ranging from chronic headaches, insomnia, and upset stomach to anxiety, depression, and high blood pressure. Because it reduces perceived stress, yoga appears to dampen the stress response. This, in turn, reduces the physiological stress response—for example, slowing the respiratory rate and lowering the heart rate and blood pressure.

In a study published in *The Journal of Alternative and Complementary Medicine,* researchers in Germany had twenty-four women take two ninety-minute yoga classes a week for three months. Women in a control group were told to maintain their normal routine.

All the women in the yoga group reported being under stress. Further, their scores for perceived stress, anxiety, and depression were higher than those of the normal population, according to the results of scientific questionnaires designed to measure these three emotional states.

At the end of the study, the yoga group reported significant improvements in their well-being. For example, their depression scores improved by 50 percent, anxiety scores by 30 percent, and their overall well-being scores by 65 percent.

You don't have to become a serious student of yoga to reap its benefits. In fact, the three poses below take just fifteen minutes, and it's likely that your stress will melt away after just a few sessions.

Practicing just three simple poses—Child's Pose, Pigeon Pose, and Seated Salutation—is enough to ease stress on a daily basis. You might also consider enrolling in a yoga class—perhaps hatha yoga, the most common form practiced in the United States. Hatha yoga combines physical poses (*asanas*), controlled breathing practiced with *asanas,* and a period of relaxation or meditation. Before you sign up for a class, observe the class once or twice to see if the style and the instructor feel right to you.

Massage

Pampering and Powerful

No matter how packed my schedule is, I always make time for a weekly full-body massage that focuses on my head and neck. (I typically hold stress and lose energy in those areas.) If you can swing it, I recommend that you do the same. We live in a pressure-cooker world, and virtually anyone would benefit from lying in a quiet, dimly lit room for forty-five minutes or so while a professional gently kneads away the tension.

What's more, studies conducted by the Touch Research Institute, part of the University of Miami School of Medicine, have found that massage slows heart rate and blood pressure and reduces levels of stress and pain hormones.

For belly pain brought on by stress, try massaging your abdomen with castor oil. It's a centuries-old remedy for nausea, pain, and cramping that I've used on my children when they have tummy problems. Lie on a thick towel while you perform this massage. While effective, this treatment can get a bit messy!

Place a quarter cup of castor oil in a small saucepan and warm on low heat for 5 minutes.

Spill Your Guts' Secrets

When my patients with IBD have flareups or experience reflux or other digestive symptoms, I always ask if stress might be a contributing factor. If they don't know—and a surprising number do not—I suggest they keep a gut diary for a short time to see if the stress in their lives coincides with their symptoms. Keeping such a diary can help you, too.

All you need is a pocket-sized notepad. A sample diary entry might look like this:

Date	Time	Stressful Event (be as specific as possible)	Stress Level (mild, moderate, severe)	Gut Symptoms	Gut Discomfort Level (mild, moderate, severe)
Monday 5/15	8:30 p.m. (after work)	Worked 12 hours today. Project due in a week; feel it won't be done. Slept poorly last night (6 hours). Skipped gym at lunch to run errands.	severe	Bloating, pain; started at 4 p.m. today.	severe

Track your digestive symptoms for a week or two. If you find that three or more "bad gut days" coincide with days of high stress, your symptoms may stem from stress. Turn down the flame of stress using the techniques in this chapter, and it's likely that your symptoms will cool down, too.

Immerse a small washcloth in the oil; wring it out very slightly.

Lying on your towel, place the oil-soaked washcloth on your belly and a heating pad set to low on top of that.

Begin to massage your belly with the tips of your fingers, using firm pressure and moving around your belly in a clockwise direction. Perform the massage for 10 minutes.

A more convenient option: the castor-oil roll-ons sold in health food stores or online. Filled with castor oil, these devices look a bit like a roll-on deodorant—simply uncap and roll the castor oil onto your abdomen.

eleven

The 21-Day Belly Fix Workout

"My reflux is unbearable," Susan said, regarding me with a mix of frustration and hope. I was her third doctor's appointment this year. The first two—both with gastroenterologists—had resulted in prescriptions for Zantac and omeprazole, the standard medications for reflux. But heartburn still kept her up at night, and she stumbled through her days, crushed by fatigue. As a high-level executive, catnaps at her desk weren't an option.

Chronic constipation was also a problem. "Right after I eat, I feel eight months pregnant," she told me. "I look it, too. I'm bloated and have gained nearly ten pounds in the past year."

I asked Susan about her diet and if she was physically active. That question hit a nerve. "I haven't worked out in two years," she said. "When I got promoted, I had to give up my yoga class—I couldn't fit it into my schedule. When I don't exercise, my diet falls apart. It's fast food when I'm busy and sweets when I'm stressed, and I'm *always* busy and stressed."

Though I could have tested Susan for a food allergy or intolerance, leaky gut, or candida, I suspected that simple lifestyle tweaks would improve her symptoms dramatically. My recommendations: Drink water throughout the day, and walk each night after work.

That was it. No prescriptions. Susan seemed surprised by that, so I expanded on my no-frills treatment. More water should alleviate the constipation, I said, and the walk would get her digestive system moving again and help cool her stress, the root of many gut-based symptoms.

At her one-month follow-up appointment, Susan was glowing. Good hydration and a regular after-work stroll had worked their digestive magic. The walk had improved her gut motility, and "going" every day was cleansing ama from her system. Her walk also eased her stress and lifted her mood. The better she felt, the better she ate—fresh, wholesome food, rather than the processed junk she'd chosen a month earlier. The five pounds she'd lost had improved her reflux so dramatically that I was able to take her off her medications. With her digestive symptoms gone, she had energy to burn in the day and slept soundly at night.

As I'd suspected, gentle, regular exercise was Susan's 21-Day Belly Fix—and it may be yours, too. In this chapter, I explain how just a little physical activity can lead to positive changes in digestive health. I also lay out the 21-Day Belly Fix Workout, which is as good for your overall health as it is for your gut.

ACTIVE BODY, HEALTHY GUT

I know it. You know it. Regular exercise does a body good. Shall we count the ways? It builds stronger, thicker bones. Improves heart and lung function. Boosts immunity. Lifts anxiety and depression. Reduces risk of heart disease, type 2 diabetes, and some cancers, including colon cancer. Builds muscle and burns fat, which helps promote a healthy weight.

Significantly, many of those benefits are linked to exercise's well-documented ability to reduce stress. Think about it. On an after-dinner stroll, the worries of the day drain away. You're mindful of the breeze on your skin, the sounds of birds or water, perhaps just the throb of your own heart. Step by step, your stress response deactivates, and your rest-and-digest response takes over. Your body releases chemicals called endorphins and may even make the neurotransmitter norepinephrine, both of which promote a feeling of well-being.

In short, one stroll rebalances mind, body, and spirit, and your gut responds positively to that inner harmony. And I haven't even gotten to the gut-specific benefits yet. Regular exercise helps the stomach empty faster, promotes proper bowel movements, and makes you sweat, which eliminates toxins through your skin. All of these actions discourage the accumulation of ama.

So many studies have associated moderate exercise with gut health, there's no room to list them all. But let me tell you about some of the most compelling findings.

- People who exercise regularly have a 40 to 50 percent lower risk of colon cancer compared with those who don't, the National Cancer Institute estimates.
- Men and women who run have a lower risk of diverticular disease than those who don't, a 2009 study published in *Medicine and Science in Sports and Exercise* found.
- In a study of people with IBS, 20–30 minutes of moderate exercise three to five times a week significantly improved volunteers' abdominal pain, stool issues, and quality of life, a 2011 study published in *The American Journal of Gastroenterology* concluded.
- Even if you're heavier than you'd like, regular exercise can help keep your gut in shape. Overweight but physically active men and women are less likely to develop stomach pain, diarrhea, and IBS than those who were not physically active, according to a 2005 study published in *Clinical Gastroenterology and Hepatology*.
- If you're a woman, moderate exercise may lower your risk of Crohn's disease by 44 percent, a 2013 analysis of physical activity involving 194,711 women published in *The British Medical Journal* found.

The upshot of these findings: If you don't have a digestive condition, regular, moderate exercise can help keep it that way. If you do, it can improve both your appetite and your mood as well as keep your symptoms at bay.

TOO MUCH OF A GOOD THING

Now that I've made the case for exercise, I'll add one important caveat: All of its benefits accrue from activity performed at a *moderate* intensity. "Moderate" in this context means that while you are exercising you can hold a conversation but are not able to sing a song.

That's good news. It means that you don't have to spend an hour on the treadmill, sweat buckets, or dread an activity that can offer both mind and body pleasure and relief from tension. When you do it properly, physical activity actually energizes you. Post-workout exhaustion is a sign of a body being pushed too hard. In fact, those who engage in extreme exercise—who run or bike long distances most days or compete in marathons—may be doing their guts more harm than good.

Day after day of intense exercise places enormous physical stress on the body and gives it too little time to rest and repair itself. The gut-brain becomes awash in adrenaline and other stress hormones, your stomach empties more slowly (ama alert!), and the lower esophageal sphincter relaxes. As you now know, this last change can lead to heartburn and GERD.

Further, if you are a long-distance runner or engage in other vigorous sports such as triathlons, you should know that cramps, bloating, diarrhea, heartburn, nausea, and gastrointestinal bleeding are common side effects. That's because extreme exercise reduces blood flow to the gut, and repeated, sustained bouncing leads to mechanical trauma. Extreme exercise can also weaken the gut lining, which raises the risk of leaky gut; unbalances the ratio of healthy and unhealthy gut bugs; and can cause gastrointestinal bleeding from lack of circulation.

Many of my patients run marathons or engage in other forms of intense physical activity because they enjoy the rush of competition. However, they don't enjoy the side effects. To heal, they must return to balance. Let me tell you about one of my patients who learned that lesson and was happier (and healthier) for it.

SHERRY'S 21-DAY BELLY FIX

Thirty-two-year-old Sherry came to my office with a grab bag of symptoms she'd struggled with for a year: a dull pain in her abdomen that seemed to get worse after meals, chronic constipation, and frequent yeast infections. She ate a healthy diet and was at a healthy weight. However, a body-composition test, which measures both lean tissue and fat tissue, revealed that Sherry was "skinny-fat"—thin, but with a high percentage of unhealthy body fat.

Her pulse was weak and hard to feel—a bad sign in both Chinese and Ayurvedic medicine. In the former, low pulse suggests qi deficiency; in the latter, weak agni. Her purple, cracked, coated tongue hinted at a stressed liver, poor digestion, and overall exhaustion. This was a woman who was pushing herself far beyond what her body could take. I just didn't know where the push was coming from.

I gathered clues as we talked about her life. At first, Sherry seemed like a typical busy mom, ping-ponging between a stressful job, her family (a handful, with three kids), and volunteer work at her church. But then she mentioned one aspect of her life that wasn't so typical: her exercise routine.

For the previous three years, Sherry had run six miles a day, virtually every day, and had competed in one marathon a year. She enjoyed the well-known "runner's high," she said. She'd also noticed that her intense runs seemed to stave off not just stress but depression, which she'd battled most of her life.

Immediately, everything clicked: Years of intense exercise—and equally intense stress—had plunged Sherry into adrenal fatigue (see chapter 3). Immediately, I put her on the 21-Day Belly Fix program and dialed down her running program—she was to run three days a week rather than five. I also recommended one session of yoga a week. Unlike running, which amps up the body's stress response, yoga activates the rest-and-digest response. Its series of postures increase blood flow to vital organs like the stomach and small intestine as it lowers the stress hormones

Kegel Your Way to a Healthy Gut

You probably know that Kegel exercises strengthen the muscles of the pelvic floor. But surprise: They also contribute to a healthy gut. In Chinese medicine, poor digestion stresses the kidney-bladder system, causing incontinence. Mainstream doctors already know that chronic constipation stresses the bladder; it obstructs the flow of urine, prevents the bladder from emptying completely, and causes the symptoms of urgency and incontinence.

Kegel exercises (also known as pelvic floor muscle exercises) strengthen the muscles under the uterus, bladder, and large intestine. If doesn't matter if you're male or female—Kegels can improve urine leakage.

When you perform Kegels, it's vital to isolate the right muscles. To find them, the next time you have to urinate, start to go, then stop. You'll feel the muscles in your vagina, bladder, or anus tighten and move up. These are the pelvic floor muscles.

Not sure whether you're tightening the right muscles? Women can place a finger into the vagina, tighten the muscles as if holding urine, and then relax them. Men can place a finger into the rectum, then imagine holding back a stream of urine. In both cases, the pelvic-floor muscles should tighten and move up and down.

Once you've isolated the pelvic-floor muscles, it's time to Kegel. To start, perform the exercise below once a day. Gradually work up to three times a day.

Empty your bladder.

Lie down or sit in a chair. Tighten the pelvic floor muscles and hold for a count of 10.

Relax the muscles completely for a count of 10.

Do 10 repetitions, 3–5 times a day. If you feel any discomfort in your abdomen or back, breathe deeply and make sure the muscles of your stomach, thighs, buttocks, and chest are relaxed.

In most cases, you'll notice improvement in four to six weeks and major improvement after three months. (So don't give up!) Further, don't over-Kegel. Increasing the number of repetitions and the frequency of exercises won't strengthen pelvic-floor muscles more quickly, and it may even fatigue the muscles and increase urine leakage.

Once you reach your goal, incorporate Kegels into your normal routine. Do a few while you brush your teeth, wait at a stoplight, or watch TV.

adrenaline and cortisol. In essence, yoga corrects hormonal imbalances and shifts the body into a mode that's more receptive to healing.

Six weeks later, I stepped into the examination room and saw a smiling Sherry. "I feel amazing," she said. Although at first she'd found it tough to cut back on her runs, she fell in love with the slow, precise postures of yoga, which helped to center her body and mind. Her abdominal pain had resolved after about three weeks, the constipation improved after just two, and the yeast infection was gone.

If Sherry's story sounds like yours, reduce your intense workouts by a third. (For example, if you exercise six days a week, drop down to four.) Then add one day of yoga or another activity that stimulate the rest-and-digest response. T'ai chi, Pilates, swimming, and walking are excellent options.

JUST RIGHT: THE 21-DAY BELLY FIX WORKOUT

To reduce stress and promote overall and digestive health, I recommend 30 minutes of light to moderate exercise most days of the week. Surprised by how little that is? Don't be. My goal is to help you feel healthier and more vibrant, not to get you ready for boot camp. Even so, don't be surprised if, after a few weeks of this workout and the 21-Day Belly Fix, you feel (and look!) lighter and leaner, with a bloat-free belly.

If you like your current workout and feel healthy and energetic, stick with it. However, if you're looking for a gentle workout that raises vitality and promotes better gut function, look no further. The 21-Day Belly Fix

Workout includes four components: walking or another form of cardio, strength training, yoga, and a core routine. Let's examine each component one by one. (Instructions and illustrations for the workouts begin on page 181.)

Walk: 20–30 minutes, most days of the week

I wish more of my patients understood that there's no need to exercise aggressively to be fit. Simply putting one foot in front of the other for 150 minutes a week—just over 20 minutes a day—can improve your health and your quality of life.

Walking is the simplest and most effective form of cardiovascular exercise there is. Like other forms of cardio, it burns calories, helps improve blood sugar, and increases gut motility and blood flow to the gut. Walking also raises your respiration and heart rate. Blood flow to the muscles and lungs increases. Small blood vessels widen to deliver more oxygen to muscles and carry away waste. Those feel-good endorphins are just a bonus.

My cardio routine couldn't be easier, gentler, or more flexible. That twenty-odd minutes a day works out to a lunchtime stroll or an after-dinner "constitutional." If walking isn't your thing, feel free to swim, ride your bicycle, hike, dig in your garden . . . any activity that raises your heart rate is fair game. If you belong to a gym, you can also spend those 150 minutes on your favorite cardio machine—spinning bike, treadmill, elliptical trainer, stair-climber, you name it.

Lift: 30 minutes, three times a week

If you are overweight, lifting weights can help you build muscle and lose fat, which will make you look better, feel better, aid blood-sugar control, and improve your health in a multitude of ways. All you need to do my simple routine is a few square feet of space, a pair of dumbbells, and a weight bench. (If you're underweight, skip this part of the workout.)

Please don't worry that strength training will bulk you up. On the contrary—as you lose fat and add dense, firm muscle, your body will look smaller. Some researchers have estimated that a pound of muscle takes up about 22 percent less space than a pound of fat!

More good news: Muscle is active tissue that gobbles calories. When you carry more lean muscle tissue, your metabolic rate can rise by as much as 15 percent. A revved-up metabolism can help make it easier to lose weight or maintain a healthy weight.

Losing excess fat also reduces the body's "burden" of toxic chemicals (such as polychlorinated biphenyls, otherwise known as PCBs), which can linger in body fat for decades.

Pose: 15 minutes, three times a week

As you've learned, I discovered the benefits of yoga in my crazy-busy twenties. Very quickly, it became my go-to exercise because it offered a good workout *and* helped me decompress from the demands of my day. I think virtually anyone can benefit from this gentle, low-impact activity.

As a yoga instructor as well as a physician, I know that the five poses in my 21-Day Belly Fix Yoga Series are among the best for digestion. They:

- increase blood flow to the digestive organs (especially the stomach and large intestine)
- increase gut motility, thereby easing constipation
- reduce inflammation and gastritis
- strengthen the small and large intestines

Yoga has also been shown to reduce stress, thereby relaxing your digestive system. And if you tend to be gassy, yoga can help with that, too.

Crunch: 15 minutes, twice a week

Your abs aren't there just to look good, and your core muscles include more than just the abs. The muscles that make up your core help support and move your spine, pelvis, rib cage, and hips, and they also play a role in

My Personal Workout

've been "on the move" all my life. As a child, I swam, biked, and even tried gymnastics and dance. Being active was a family affair, too, although back then, I didn't "exercise." I had fun in the pool or on the basketball court with my mom, dad, and sisters.

Being active became more important in college and medical school. After hours of study in the library, every muscle in my body was itching to move. Abandoning my books, I'd hit the gym to lift weights or use the cardio machines, or I'd run along one of the quiet roads around the campus.

I discovered yoga and Pilates in my late twenties, after my residency. They quickly became my favorite forms of exercise; both activities relaxed my mind and strengthened muscles that running simply didn't touch. As I've mentioned, I even became a certified yoga teacher because I predicted that I'd be far too busy later in life to make it to regular classes. (That surely turned out to be true!)

Today, exercise is absolutely vital for my mental and emotional health. As a physician, I spend so much time in my head that exercise re-grounds me. I try to work out for at least forty minutes three or four days a week, either at my home gym or the gym where my family and I are members. I do it all—Pilates, swimming, cardio machines—and every three weeks, I switch up my routine. Once a week, I practice *vinyasa* flow yoga at home. It's challenging (it involves headstands!), but for me it's ninety minutes of pure relaxation.

Given my schedule, I've had to let go of my former all-or-nothing mentality, where if I don't work out for at least an hour it's not worth it. Instead, I do what I can, when I can. If I am traveling, I walk the city I'm in or use the gym at my hotel. At home, there are more options—my home gym, the local gym my family belongs to, the parks in the city. And just as I was active with my family, Vik and I now take our children to play tennis, shoot hoops, or swim laps at the pool. For them, it isn't "exercise"—it's having fun with Mom and Dad. And that's good, because moving your body, just for the joy of it, is one of life's simple pleasures.

a healthy digestive system. Performing this simple core routine a few times a week will help:

- tone the muscles of your midsection
- train the muscles in your lower back, hips, and abdomen to work together
- increase digestive blood flow
- loosen trigger points in the bowel wall, easing abdominal pain from constipation, diverticulosis, and poor gut motility
- reduce the pressure of excess belly fat on the abdominal wall, which can help to reduce reflux and improve GERD symptoms
- improve balance (it's all about balance, one way or another!)

The 21-Day Belly Fix Core Routine includes a classic move from Pilates called "The 100," along with other research-tested exercises that will tone and tighten as they promote digestion. Choose 2–3 different core exercises from the series and perform 3–4 sets of 10–12 reps each.

PUTTING YOUR 21-DAY BELLY FIX WORKOUT TO WORK

Here's what a week of the 21-Day Belly Fix Workout might look like. Feel free to follow it as shown or rearrange it to suit your schedule. With this program, *you* get to decide what's on your workout "menu." That's by design. When you make your workout *yours,* it becomes an automatic part of your day that you won't want to miss!

Monday	Tuesday	Wednesday	Thursday	Friday	Saturday	Sunday
Cardio, 20–30 minutes; strength training		Cardio, 20–30 minutes; strength training		Cardio, 20–30 minutes; strength training	30-minute walk	30-minute walk
		21-Day Belly Fix Core Routine			21-Day Belly Fix Core Routine	

	21-Day Belly Fix Yoga Series		21-Day Belly Fix Yoga Series			21-Day Belly Fix Yoga Series

NOTE: "CARDIO" HERE IS DEFINED AS WALKING, SWIMMING, BICYCLING, TENNIS, JOGGING AND CYCLING, AS WELL AS USING MACHINES LIKE ELLIPTICAL TRAINERS AND TREADMILLS.

KEEP YOUR 21-DAY BELLY FIX GOING

Once you're in the exercise groove, you'll be amazed at how your mood and energy soar. If you're anything like my patients, you'll look forward to moving your body each day! Even so, there are a number of ways to maximize this workout's benefits and keep your motivation strong.

SWITCH THINGS UP. Every three weeks, change up your workout. If you walk, explore different terrains (dirt instead of asphalt) or add different routes that include hills. Or give walking a break and hit the pool at your gym or enroll in a t'ai chi or Pilates class. Build on the strength-training moves, yoga poses, or core exercises in this book. Varying your exercise routines challenges your body, works all of your muscle groups, and keep your motivation high.

ADD "BURSTS" TO A BUSY DAY. On days when you don't have time for your regular walk or workout, add three 10-minute bursts of exercise to your day. University of Virginia researchers had middle-aged men and women complete fifteen 10-minute exercise routines a week. In just three weeks, they showed a 10 to 15 percent improvement in aerobic fitness; an increase in strength and muscular endurance from 40 percent to 100 percent; and a 15-point drop in total cholesterol.

While you can "burst" at home, the office is a great place to sneak in a 10-minute workout; you can fit in your 30 minutes and reduce stress at the same time. Any activity will do—the point is to move. Trot up and down a flight of stairs. Walk around the block. If you work at home, put a rebounder in your office and bounce between e-mails. During housework, break out your MP3 player and start an impromptu dance party for one. Or simply do a few sets of jumping jacks.

USE YOUR SMART PHONE TO SCHEDULE YOUR WORKOUTS. Our tablets and smart phones may have a tendency to keep us on the couch, but they can also help you get off it. Put your workouts on your phone calendar, along with your appointments at the doctor, hair salon, or vet. When exercise is scheduled, you don't have to "find the time." You've already found it!

RELAX AND ENJOY. Haven't exercised in a while? Don't let that throw you. Focus on health and stress management and let your weight take care of itself. And it will, if you come to see your workout as a gift that you give to yourself. Feeling good about where you are *right now* will keep you in balance and on the path to health and vitality.

twelve

The Alternative Therapies

At the start of this book, I said that you don't need a doctor to give you a 21-Day Belly Fix—truly, this is a DIY program! Many of my patients need no more than the program in this book to heal.

However, those diagnosed with a functional gut disorder such as IBS or IBD, chronic health conditions such as allergies or GERD, or psychological issues such as anxiety and depression need a few more tools in their gut-repair kits, and you may, too. That's why I wrote this section, which offers alternative therapies not included in the 21-Day Belly Fix program.

These are the therapies my patients ask about the most, the ones that their other doctors have recommended as part of their treatment plans. I've used several of them myself or to treat my patients. Several, it must be said, may seem kind of "out there." For example, most mainstream doctors dismiss hypnotherapy, commonly known as hypnotism, as little more than a side-show attraction. But the fact is, the National Institutes of Health (NIH) has recommended hypnotherapy as a treatment for chronic pain for twenty years, and I've used hypnosis to treat gut pain rooted in emotional trauma and abuse.

As you read this chapter, keep an open mind and give these therapies a fair shake. Some, such as gut-directed hypnotherapy, have been rigorously tested in clinical studies. Others, such as Epsom salt baths and homeopathy, have been used to treat gut-based symptoms for hundreds or even thousands of years.

All but the first two therapies require you to work with an experienced practitioner trained to administer the therapy in question; that person will partner with your primary-care doctor or health-care team. If you consider adding any of these therapies to your treatment plan, please do your research as you select a practitioner. Where possible, I provide links to the appropriate licensing bodies.

HOME TREATMENTS TO TRY

Abdominal Cramping and Constipation

Magnesium Supplements, Soaks, or Oil

The mineral magnesium is nature's muscle relaxant. It plays an important role in muscle contraction and relaxation. You know this if you've ever soaked in a tub to which you've added Epsom salts, which are pure magnesium sulfate. Magnesium's relaxing effect extends to the muscles of the colon, so if you're chronically constipated, this mineral can loosen things up. Magnesium supplements, Epsom salt baths, and magnesium oil can all relieve abdominal cramping and constipation. However, it's vital to use the form that's right for you, especially if diarrhea is one of your primary symptoms.

I test my patients for magnesium deficiency because many have been diagnosed with conditions that can deplete magnesium in the body, including IBS, IBD, type 2 diabetes, hyperthyroidism, and kidney disease. Chronic stress, heavy menstrual flow, and the use of diuretics (common in patients with high blood pressure, heart disease, and hormone imbalances) also can deplete the body of magnesium. Although some of the symptoms of magnesium deficiency are physical—nausea and vomiting, restless legs syndrome, abnormal heart rhythms, low blood pressure—a deficiency can also cause anxiety, confusion, and insomnia.

When a blood test reveals that a patient is magnesium-deficient and diarrhea is not a problem for them, I recommend an oral supplement—magnesium in its chelated form. "Chelated" minerals bond to protein molecules, which carry them to the bloodstream and thereby improve their absorption. (Other forms of magnesium have poor bioavailability, meaning that they are hard for the body to use.)

However, magnesium taken in supplement form can cause abdominal cramping and diarrhea because this mineral stimulates intestinal motility. (I told you: Magnesium is nature's muscle relaxant!) Ditto if you take certain medications—oral magnesium supplements can interact with a wide variety of prescription drugs, including antibiotics and blood pressure medications.

To ensure that your system tolerates oral magnesium, begin with a low dose—100 milligrams, taken at night. After a night or two, if all goes well, increase to 200 milligrams and then 400 milligrams.

If any of these low doses cause abdominal cramping or diarrhea, switch to a form of magnesium that is absorbed through the skin. You have two choices: a good old-fashioned bath in Epsom salts or a magnesium-oil massage.

If you opt for the bath (which I highly recommend—it's very soothing!), add two cups of Epsom salts to a warm tub and soak for at least fifteen minutes three times a week. Less magnesium is absorbed through the skin, which means you will get enough of the mineral to relieve constipation and cramps but not enough to cause diarrhea. For a treat, stir in 5–10 drops of essential oil along with the Epsom salts. Essential oils of lavender, rose, bergamot, or jasmine can help relax you, while essential oils of peppermint, rosemary, or eucalyptus will invigorate you.

Magnesium oil, available in health food stores, is another option. To promote proper elimination, massage one tablespoon into the soles of your feet and into your abdomen each night before bed.

Nausea and Heartburn

Ginger Lozenges

Many of my patients notice that their digestive symptoms are worse in the morning, and sometimes their days begin with nausea that takes hours to resolve. (If you recall, that's exactly what happened to my husband, Vik.) Often, this morning nausea is a clue that they need a 21-Day Belly Fix. But while we work on gut renovation, ginger lozenges can help relieve those waves of nausea that come and go with no warning. (As you may know, ginger also relieves the nausea associated with early pregnancy or seasickness as well as the queasiness that can accompany migraines and the nausea caused by chemotherapy.)

Practitioners of Chinese and Ayurvedic medicine have used ginger to treat ailments as diverse as colds, arthritis, migraines, and hypertension for thousands of years. However, this medicinal herb is especially valued for its ability to ease digestive upset. Research suggests that ginger improves gut motility, increases the production of stomach acid, and regulates the production and passing of intestinal gas. It's thought that a substance called gingerol, abundant in fresh ginger and responsible for the root's spicy fragrance, is the main ingredient behind ginger's belly-friendly pharmacological and physiological effects.

If you are having a particularly bad belly day, with lots of nausea or heartburn, pop a ginger lozenge, available in health food stores, three times a day. Select a brand that contains gingerol—I'd recommend a particular brand, but as long as they contain gingerol, they're all effective.

If you don't care for lozenges, sip a cup of ginger tea. Or do as I do when my belly is upset: Grate a teaspoon of fresh root, stir into a cup of boiling water, and let steep for five minutes. It's warming, spicy, and delicious.

WHAT A DOCTOR CAN DO

Indigestion and Nausea

Homeopathy

Developed in Germany at the end of the eighteenth century, homeopathy is rooted in two theories. The first is that "like cures like"—disease can be cured by a substance that produces similar symptoms in healthy people. The second theory, the "law of minimum dose," asserts that the *lower* the dose of the substance, the *greater* its effectiveness.

Homeopathic remedies are made from substances found in plants, minerals, or animals, from red onion and arnica (mountain herb) to crushed whole bees and stinging nettle. My mother-in-law, an Ayurvedic physician in India, was the first to turn me on to homeopathy. Today, two of my "go-to" homeopathic treatments for gut distress are *Chelidonium majus,* which can ease indigestion and nausea and help detoxify the liver, and *Nux Vomica,* which helps ease symptoms of indigestion and nausea. (Vik recalls his mother dosing him *Nux Vomica* to help calm his gastrointestinal distress.)

Homeopathic remedies are often formulated as ointments, gels, drops, creams, tablets, or sugar pellets to be placed under the tongue. It is not uncommon for different people with the same condition to receive different treatments. Most practitioners, myself included, tailor remedies to each person, often considering his or her history of disease, symptoms, complexion, and pulse.

While mainstream physicians debate the efficacy of homeopathy, it is widely accepted throughout Europe and Asia. However, because homeopathic remedies can interact with other supplements or medications, it's important to use homeopathic remedies only under the supervision of an experienced practitioner. Laws regulating the practice of homeopathy in the United States vary from state to state. Select a practitioner who has been certified by one of several organizations: the National Board of Homeopathic Examiners (www.nbhe.org), the Council for Homeopathic

Certification (www.homeopathicdirectory.com), or the North American Society for Homeopaths (www.homeopathy.org).

IBS and Gut Troubles Rooted in Trauma

Gut-Directed Hypnotherapy

When you have a belly issue, the pain and discomfort are real. However, gut dysfunction can also be a physical expression of emotional, sexual, or physical trauma that has been repressed by the unconscious mind. This repressed emotional pain finds expression in physical symptoms. (This is especially true of children and teens.) In these types of cases, hypnosis can offer significant and dramatic relief.

At your first visit, a hypnotherapist will take your medical history, ask what condition brought you in, and explain what hypnosis is and how it works. Then, he or she will direct you through some relaxation techniques, using a series of mental images and suggestions intended to change behaviors and relieve symptoms. For example, a hypnotherapist may suggest that people who suffer with chronic constipation visualize their bowels as a river and that the current is gradually picking up speed. Typically, a hypnotherapist will also teach you the basics of self-hypnosis and give you an audiotape to use at home so that you can reinforce what you learn during the session.

A specialized form of hypnosis, called gut-directed hypnotherapy, has been found to relieve the symptoms of adults with abdominal pain and IBS. Gut-directed hypnotherapy uses hypnotic induction with progressive relaxation and other techniques, followed by imagery directed at the gut. Multiple reviews of the research have shown that it may be helpful in managing IBS symptoms. Several studies of hypnotherapy for IBS have shown substantial long-term improvement of gastrointestinal symptoms as well as anxiety, depression, disability, and quality of life.

For example, in a 2012 study published in *The American Journal of Gastroenterology,* people with severe IBS received one 60-minute hypnotherapy session a week for three months. The sessions were held at either psychologists' private offices or at a small county hospital. Control groups received information on IBS physiology, diet, and/or relaxation techniques.

Those who underwent hypnosis reported significantly reduced symptoms, reduced anxiety, and improved quality of life. Best of all, the therapy worked at both specialized research centers and common health-care settings that the typical patient would use. The control groups experienced no significant improvement.

Best of all, the benefits of gut-directed hypnotherapy seem to last. The results seen at 3 months were sustained up to 1 year.

Each hypnotherapy session lasts about an hour, and most people start to see results within 4–10 sessions. To find licensed health professionals who practice hypnosis, log onto the American Society of Clinical Hypnosis (www.asch.net) or the Societies of Hypnosis (www.SocietiesOfHypnosis .com).

Abdominal Pain Caused by Underlying Trauma

Marma Therapy

This therapy is one of several forms of *energy healing,* which involves the transfer of healing energy through the hands of a practitioner into another's body to rebalance its energy and restore health. Wacky? Hardly. Many, many of my patients use energy healing in their treatment plans. Further, marma is the Ayurvedic "twist" on energy healing, and—like Reiki from Japan and qigong from China—has a long and venerable tradition.

In Ayurvedic literature, the word *marma* comes from the root *varman,* which means vital or hidden energy point. Marma therapy, then, is the healing art of balancing the chakras and therefore the body's flow of energy. Marma involves stimulating "marma points"—similar to acupressure points—with vigorous pressure to promote healing. There are 107 marma points where flesh, veins, arteries, tendons, bones, and joints meet, and it is believed that marma's effectiveness is related to the sensitivity of these points.

I have a wonderful woman in my practice who offers marma therapy, and I've experienced it myself—it's intensely relaxing. In general, you disrobe to your skivvies and lie under a sheet. The practitioner first identifies the chakra imbalance and massages the corresponding points with essential oils. He or she typically also uses a sound tuning instrument to ground and enhance your breathing, and placed gemstones or rocks that correspond to the chakras to stimulate key marma points. In my practice, I have seen chronic constipation, functional abdominal pain, and IBS relieved with marma therapy; patients leave feeling more relaxed, and with less gut discomfort.

In my experience, energy healing in general, and marma in particular, works best for those with stress or unresolved traumas. Marma restores balance to the nervous system, gets rids of toxins at a cellular level, and helps the brain release of neurotransmitters that affect mood and pain. It promotes an overall feeling of rejuvenation and brings body, mind, and spirit into harmony.

Marma therapy is rather new to the United States, so there is currently no licensing body. My advice: Search for a practitioner who has education and training in Ayurvedic medicine and who is familiar with this therapy.

Gut Issues Rooted in Stress or Trauma

Craniosacral Therapy

My job requires me to expend enormous amounts of emotional and mental energy. At times, I must bear and absorb the pain and trauma some of my patients have experienced. As a healer, I am honored to be called on to absorb this pain. However, it does affect my own energy levels. In my integrative fellowship, my colleagues and I were taught that we must find a way to "off-load" this negative energy, lest it affect our own health.

Craniosacral therapy is my way; I treat myself to it once or twice a month. After a session, I can literally feel the energy and vitality returning to my mind and brain. I feel invigorated and think more clearly. This alternative therapy is used to treat a wide variety of health issues, including

Hypnosis Can Heal a Traumatized Gut

While I am not a licensed hypnotist, I have been trained in this modality and have used it on my patients. I recall a patient in her mid-twenties who came to my office with recurrent abdominal pain and bloating. Her symptoms began in high school and persisted through her college years, affecting her grades and school success. At her first visit, she revealed that her childhood had been filled with chaos and abuse but added that she thought she was "over it."

I recommended several sessions of hypnosis. During our sessions, I learned that she had been physically abused and that her abuser had hit her in the stomach multiple times. I taught her to reframe her memories so that they were not as emotionally intrusive. After three sessions, she noticed that she did, indeed, have less belly pain and fewer episodes of bloating.

At this point, I referred her to a licensed hypnotist for further work. Our few sessions had shown her that she had not been over the abuse—her gut had merely "told" her so.

migraines, autism, fibromyalgia, and chronic pain. In my experience, this modality also helps to heal gut issues rooted in stress and trauma, including functional abdominal pain, IBS, and chronic constipation or diarrhea. Just one session can clear or unblock stuck digestive energy, opening the body to the potential of healing.

Craniosacral therapy is an offshoot of osteopathy, which emphasizes the role of the musculoskeletal system in health and disease. It evaluates and enhances the function of the *craniosacral system,* which is made up of the membranes and cerebrospinal fluid that surround and protect the brain and spinal cord. The goal of craniosacral therapy is to release restrictions in this system to improve central nervous system function.

In a typical session, which lasts 30–90 minutes, you sit and then lie quietly, fully clothed, while the practitioner exerts gentle finger pressure at points around your head, feet, or sacrum (the triangular bone at the bottom of the spine). Unlike, say, chiropractic therapy, there is no wrenching of the neck or spine.

When selecting a practitioner, it is important to find someone with whom you feel comfortable and safe. To begin your search, log onto the Biodynamic Craniosacral Therapy Association of North America (www .craniosacraltherapy.org) or the Upledger Institute (www.upledger.com.)

Exercises and Yoga

To perform the stress-management exercises in chapter 10 and the 21-Day Belly Fix Workout in chapter 11, you'll need the following equipment:

- Yoga mat or thick towel or blanket
- Flat weight bench
- 5- and 8-pound dumbbells (you can add 10- and 15-pound weights as your fitness level increases)

YOGA FOR STRESS MANAGEMENT

Mountain Pose

Often the beginning of a yoga series, Mountain Pose is meant to ground your life energy so that you feel as stable and immovable as a mountain. In stressful times, grounding energy is essential.

1. Stand straight with your feet together, distributing your weight evenly over both feet. Spread your toes like a fan.

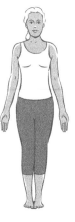

2. Tighten your thighs so that your knee muscles lift and tuck in your tailbone.

3. Straighten your arms, with your palms facing forward.

4. Pull your shoulder blades back and lift your chest.

5. Look straight ahead. Hold the pose for 1 or 2 minutes.

Tree Pose

The challenge of this pose is to force the restless mind to focus on staying in balance—quite literally. Should your mind wander to your to-do list, you will topple!

1. Stand with your feet together. Lifting your arms, press your palms together as if praying, and hold them in front of your chest.

2. Lift your right foot off the ground, turn your right knee out to the side, and place the sole of your right foot on the inside of your left leg. Your right heel should be just above your left knee. Hold for 2 breaths.

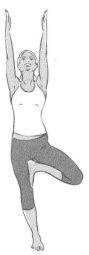

3. Lift your right foot from your left leg; grasp it with your right hand. Using your hand, position your right foot on the inside of your left leg, with your right heel just below your groin. The sole of your right foot should gently press into your left thigh. Return hands to prayer position. Hold for 3 to 5 breaths.

4. Release your right foot from your left leg, turn your right knee to point straight in front of you, and lower your foot to the floor.

5. Lower your hands to your sides. Repeat with your other leg, lifting your left foot off the ground.

Corpse Pose

A bit creepy-sounding, but this pose can relax your body and your mind as well as activate the sympathetic nervous system. And how often do you lie still when you're stressed? Now is your opportunity.

1. Sit on the floor with your knees bent and your feet on the floor. Lean back onto your forearms.
2. Slowly extend your right leg, then your left, pushing through your heels.
3. Release both legs, letting your feet drop to either side.
4. Lie back, resting your arms at your sides. Then turn your arms outward, resting the backs of your hands on your mat.
5. Close your eyes. Hold the pose 5 to 10 minutes.

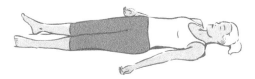

Prayer Pose

This pose is a chance to connect—with yourself, your Higher Power, or any other source of spiritual sustenance.

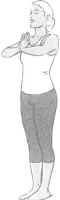

1. Stand with your arms at your sides and your heels together, placing your weight on the balls of your feet. Stand as tall as possible. Lift your chest and draw your shoulders down and back.
2. Lifting your arms, press your palms together over your breastbone. Relax your mind and fix your eyes on object in front of you.
3. Hold this position for one minute, breathing normally.

THE 21-DAY BELLY FIX STRENGTH TRAINING WORKOUT

For all of these exercises, perform three sets of 10–12 repetitions. When you can perform three sets with ease and good form, move up to slightly heavier dumbbells.

Dumbbell Woodchops

A great warm-up exercise, woodchops target your entire core, including your obliques (which run down your sides) and abdominal muscles.

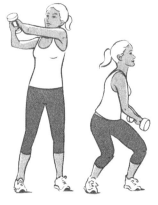

1. Hold one dumbbell in both hands, arms at your sides. Stand with your feet slightly wider than shoulder-width apart.
2. Slowly and with control, swing the dumbbell up and across your body and over your opposite shoulder. Then swing it back down to your hip, with the same control.

Dumbbell Front Squat

This exercise targets muscles in your back, butt, and hips. Contract your abdominal muscles throughout the exercise—this stabilizes your back.

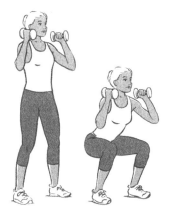

1. Hold a dumbbell in each hand, arms at your sides, palms facing inward. Stand with your feet slightly wider than hip-width apart and turned slightly outward. Pull your shoulder blades down and back. Contract your abdominal muscles.

2. Bring the dumbbells to just in front of your shoulders. Keep your chest lifted and your chin slightly lifted. Shift your weight into your heels.

3. *Downward phase.* Bend your knees and slowly shift forward until your thighs are parallel or almost parallel to the floor. In this lowered position, keep your feet firmly planted and your weight evenly distributed between the balls and heels of both feet. Don't let your knees travel too far past your toes, and do not tuck or arch your lower back.

4. *Upward phase.* Keeping your back, chest, and head lifted, exhale and return to start position by pushing your feet into the floor through your heels. Your hips and torso should rise together, and your knees should line up with your second toe.

Dumbbell Step-Up

This exercise will give your butt and thighs a good workout. Throughout this exercise, work to keep your knee aligned over your second toe and also to keep your ankles straight (don't let them collapse in or out).

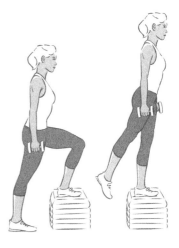

1. Stand with your feet about hip width apart; hold dumbbells with palms facing in. Pull your shoulders down and back. Try not to shrug your shoulder upward.

2. *Upward phase.* Slowly step up to place your *right* foot firmly on the platform, keeping your torso upright and aligning your knee over your second toe. Push off with your *left* leg to raise your body onto the platform, placing your left foot alongside your right.

3. *Downward phase.* Leaning slightly forward, slowly load your weight onto your *right* foot, stepping backward to place your *left* foot on the floor in its starting position. Then switch feet and load

your weight into your *left* foot and step off the platform with your *right* foot, returning to starting position.

Dumbbell Bench Press

This exercise will firm and shape your arms, chest, and shoulders. Throughout this exercise, make sure that your head, shoulders, and butt make contact with the bench and that your feet make contact with the floor.

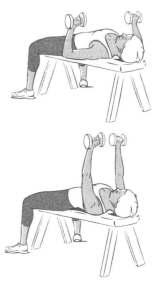

1. Lie on your back on a flat bench with your feet planted firmly on the floor and your spine in a neutral position. Grasp a dumbbell in each hand, palms facing forward.
2. Pull your shoulder blades down and back so that they make firm contact with the bench. Keeping your wrists in neutral, press the dumbbells toward the ceiling until they're directly above your breastbone. Your arms should be fully extended and your wrists straight.
3. *Downward phase.* Inhale. In a slow and controlled manner, lower the dumbbells in unison until they are almost level with your midchest. Keeping your wrists straight, gently touch the dumbbells to your chest without bouncing.
4. Pause, then press the dumbbells back to the starting position.

Lying Dumbbell Pec Fly

This exercise targets muscles in your chest and shoulders. Throughout the exercise, make sure that your shoulders and butt make constant contact with the bench and that your feet are planted firmly on the floor.

1. Lie on your back on a flat bench, planting your feet on the floor. From a lying position, grasp each dumbbell with your palms fac-

ing forward and your thumbs wrapped around the handle.

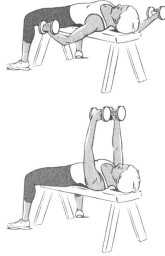

2. Pull your shoulder blades down and back so that they make firm contact with the bench. Now, lift the dumbbells to a position shoulder-width apart, keeping your elbows almost straight and your wrists straight (the "neutral" position). Turn your arms so that your palms face inward.

3. *Downward phase.* Inhale and, slowly and with control, lower the dumb-bells in a wide arc until they are level with your shoulders or chest. Keep the dumbbells parallel during the movement. Remember to keep your elbows slightly bent and your wrists straight.

4. *Upward phase.* Keeping your elbows and wrists in the neutral po-sition, exhale as you slowly return the dumbbells toward the ceil-ing in a wide arc.

Dumbbell Lateral Raise

This move can help give you firm, shapely shoulders. Contract your abdominal mus-cles and pull your shoulder blades down and back throughout the exercise.

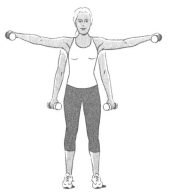

1. Stand with your feet slightly wider than hip-width apart. Hold the dumbbells at your sides, thumbs wrapped around the dumbbell handles, palms facing your body, elbows relaxed. Contract your abdominal muscles and pull your shoulder blades down and back. Align your head and neck with your spine.

2. *Upward phase.* Exhale and, slowly and with control, raise the dumbbells up and out to your sides. Let your elbows and upper arms rise together and lead the movement ahead of your forearms and dumbbells. As your arms near shoulder level, turn your thumbs slightly upward. Continue raising the dumbbells until your arms are level with your shoulders and approximately parallel with the floor. Keep your torso erect and your wrists straight.

3. *Downward phase.* Inhale and, slowly and with control, gently lower the dumbbells to starting position, keeping your elbows almost straight. As you lower the dumbbells, rotate your thumbs slightly downward.

THE 21-DAY BELLY FIX YOGA DIGESTIVE SERIES

Downward Dog

The essential yoga pose, Downward Dog stretches almost every muscle in the body, while massaging the internal organs, especially those in the abdomen.

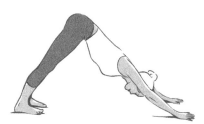

1. Get on your hands and knees on your mat. Align your knees directly below your hips and place your hands, palms down, 6 to 12 inches in front of your shoulders. Place your index fingers side by side and turn your toes under.

2. Exhale and, pushing with your palms, lift your knees off the mat. Lift your sit bones (the bones under the flesh of your butt) toward the ceiling and push the top of your thighs back so that your body looks like an inverted "V." At first, keep your knees slightly bent and your heels lifted away from the mat.

3. With an exhalation, push the tops of your thighs back and stretch your heels onto or down toward the floor. Straighten your knees, but be sure not to lock them. Firm the outer thighs and

roll the upper thighs inward slightly. Narrow the front of the pelvis.

4. Gently begin to move your chest back toward your thighs until your ears are even with your upper arms. Keep your head between your upper arms; don't let it hang.

5. Keep your hips lifting and push strongly into your hands. Stay in this pose for 1–3 minutes. Then bend your knees to the floor with an exhalation and rest in Child's Pose (next pose).

Child's Pose

This pose indirectly massages the abdominal wall, which stimulates gut motility.

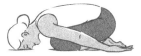

1. Kneel on your mat. Sit on your heels, with your big toes touching, then separate your knees to about hip-width apart. Place your hands on your thighs.

2. Exhale and bring your torso down between your thighs until your chest is resting on your thighs and your forehead is resting on the mat.

3. Place your hands on the floor alongside your torso, palms up, and release the fronts of your shoulders toward the floor. Feel how the weight of the front shoulders pulls the shoulder blades wide across your back.

4. Stay in this position anywhere from 30 seconds to a few minutes.

Happy Baby Pose

I love this pose! Lying on your back opens your pelvis, thereby activating the liver and gallbladder.

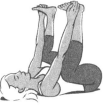

1. Lie on your back on the mat, with knees bent, feet flat on the floor about hip-width apart, arms alongside the body, palms facing the ceiling.

2. Exhale, then lift your feet off the mat and bend your knees toward your shoulders.

3. Inhale, grasping the outsides of your feet with your hands. Open your knees slightly, then raise them up toward your armpits. Your ankles should be directly over your knees, so that your shins are perpendicular to the floor.

4. Gently push your feet up into your hands as you pull your hands down to create resistance.

5. Press your tailbone into the mat and lengthen the base of your skull away from the back of your neck.

6. Hold the pose for 30–60 seconds.

Seated Forward Bend

Here's another pose that massages the abdomen.

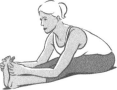

1. Sit on the edge of your yoga mat with your legs extended. Reach actively through your heels. Inhale as you reach your arms out to the side and then over your head, lengthening your spine.

2. Exhaling, bend forward from your hips (not your waist) as you lengthen the front of your torso. Imagine your torso coming to rest on your thighs, instead of tipping your nose toward your knees.

3. Depending on your degree of flexibility, grasp your shins, ankles, or feet.

4. Keep the front of your torso straight; do not round your back. Let your belly touch your legs first, then your chest, and finally your head and nose.

5. Hold for up to 1 minute. With each inhalation, lengthen the front torso. With each exhalation, fold a bit deeper.

6. To release the pose, draw your tailbone toward the floor as you inhale and lift your torso.

Seated Twist

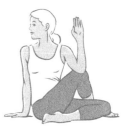

Twisting poses like this one are thought to improve elimination by activating both the small and large intestines.

1. Sit on the floor with your spine straight and your legs stretched out in front of you.
2. Bend your left leg to bring your left foot over your right knee. Place your left foot on the floor.
3. Inhale deeply as you face forward, then slowly twist your upper back to your left as you exhale.
4. Hold this position for 10 seconds.
5. Inhale as you release to face back to the front.
6. Repeat on the other side.

THE 21-DAY BELLY FIX CORE WORKOUT

The 100

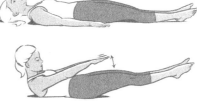

Often considered a warm-up exercise, this classic Pilates move is the ultimate core workout. To do it correctly, you must coordinate your breath with the movement.

1. Lie flat on a mat with your legs squeezed together, arms by your side.
2. Contract your abdominals, squeeze your buttocks, and lift both legs a few inches off the mat. As you lift, make sure you can feel the lift coming from those muscles.
3. Raise your arms, reach them forward over your thighs and pump them up and down. Inhale deeply and steadily as you pump your

arms up and down five times, then exhale and pump five more times.

4. A set equals 10 pumps. Work up to doing ten consecutive sets, which equals 100 pumps.

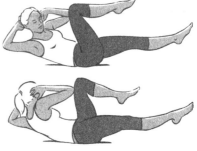

Crunches

As you perform this exercise, focus on contracting your abdominals. Proper breathing is important, too— exhale as you curl up, inhale as you lower back down.

1. Lie on your back on a mat with your knees bent, feet flat on the floor, and heels 12–18 inches from your butt.
2. Place your hands behind your head. Pull your shoulder blades to- gether and your elbows back without arching your low back. Maintain this elbow position throughout the exercise. Your head should be aligned with your spine.
3. Contract your abdominal and core muscles to stabilize your spine. Nod your chin slightly as you slowly curl your head and shoulders off the mat. Keep your neck relaxed and your feet and tailbone in contact with the mat at all times. Do not pull forward on your head. Continue curling up until your upper back is lifted off the mat. Hold this position briefly.
4. Gently inhale as you lower your torso back toward the mat slowly and with control. Keep your feet, tailbone and low back in contact with the mat.

Plank Pose

Simple, yet challenging, the plank is a classic core exercise. If you experi- ence any pain in your lower back with this movement, however, stop right away.

1. On your mat, lie on your stomach, elbows close to your sides
and directly under your shoulders, palms down and fingers
facing forward. Contract your
abdominal and core muscles.
Contract your thigh muscles to
straighten your legs and flex
your ankles, tucking your toes
toward your shins.

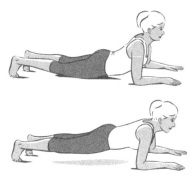

2. Slowly lift your torso and thighs off the mat. Keep your torso and
legs rigid. Do not allow your lower back or ribs to sag. Avoid lifting your hips into the air or bending your knees. Keep the shoulders away from the ears (no shrugging). Your shoulders should be
directly over your elbows with your palms facing down through
the entire exercise. Hold this position for at least 5 seconds, continuing to breathe and keeping the abdominals strong.

3. Keep your torso and legs stiff as you slowly and gently lower your
body back toward the mat.

The Bicycle

Perform this exercise slowly and with control. Do not pull forward on
your head. During the upward and downward movement of your trunk,
it is important to keep your lower back pressed into the floor or mat.

1. On your mat, lie on your
back with your knees bent,
your feet flat on the mat,
your hands behind your
head, and your elbows point-
ing out to the sides. Contract
your abdominal muscles and
lift both feet off the mat.

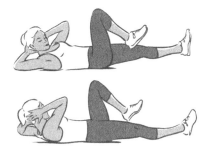

2. Extend your left leg while drawing your right knee toward your chest. At the same time, raise your shoulders off the floor, and bring your left shoulder across your body toward your right knee. Don't pull on your neck. Pause, then switch sides. Repeat, alternating sides throughout the exercise.

Recipes

SMOOTHIES

Blueberry Pie

MAKES 1 SERVING

½ cup frozen unsweetened wild blueberries
Juice of ½ lemon
1 scoop vanilla protein powder
½ cup water
½ cup ice

Blend all ingredients until thoroughly combined.

Per serving: 180 calories, 15.41 g protein, 3.56 g fat (.31 saturated), 22.09 g carbohydrates, 9.15 g sugars, 8.2 g fiber, 131 mg sodium

Banana Chocolate

MAKES 1 SERVING

1 medium banana, frozen
1 scoop chocolate protein powder
1 cup water

Blend all ingredients until thoroughly combined, adding water until desired consistency is reached.

Per serving: 256 calories, 17.37 g protein, 5.35 g fat (.44 saturated), 39.61 g carbohydrates, 16.43 g sugars, 9.2 g fiber, 141 mg sodium

Berry Blast

MAKES 1 SERVING

1 cup unsweetened frozen strawberries
½ medium avocado
1 scoop plain protein powder
½ cup ice cubes
Water as needed

Blend all ingredients until thoroughly combined, adding water until desired consistency is reached.

Per serving: 289 calories, 16.97 g protein, 13.64 g fat (1.76 saturated), 15.45 g carbohydrates, 15.45 g sugars, 13.7 g fiber, 138 mg sodium

Vanilla Date

MAKES 1 SERVING

1 Medjool date, pit removed
½ medium banana, frozen

1 scoop vanilla protein powder

1 cup water

Blend all ingredients until thoroughly combined, adding water until desired consistency is reached.

Per serving: 254 calories, 16.07 g protein, 3.23 g fat (.37 saturated), 42.47 g carbohydrates, 25.17 g sugars, 9.10 g fiber, 131 mg sodium

Tropical Colada

MAKES 1 SERVING

½ cup frozen mango chunks

½ cup cubed pineapple

1 scoop tropical or plain flavored protein powder

½ cup ice cubes

⅓ cup water

Blend all ingredients until thoroughly combined.

Per serving: 214 calories, 16.13 g protein, 3.41 g fat (.38 saturated), 31.78 g carbohydrates, 21.40 g sugars, 8.5 g fiber, 132 mg sodium

DR. TAZ'S GREEN JUICE BLENDS

The Refreshing One

MAKES 1 SERVING

½ medium apple

½ medium ripe pear

1 medium cucumber

¾ cup chopped kale

½ lemon, seeds removed

Chop the apple, pear, and cucumber. Add all ingredients to blender and pulse, adding water to thin as needed.

Per serving: 173 calories, 4.71 g protein, 1.08 g fat (.45 saturated), 43.11 g carbohydrates, 25.07 g sugars, 8.4 g fiber, 27 mg sodium

The Savory One

MAKES 1 SERVING

3 leaves romaine lettuce
1 celery stalk
2 kale leaves
½ large apple
¼ lemon, seeds removed
½ teaspoon grated ginger
½ cup water

Chop the lettuce, celery, kale, and apple. Add ingredients to blender and pulse until combined.

Per serving: 89 calories, 3.08 g protein, .85 g fat (.17 saturated), 21.29 g carbohydrates, 19.63 g sugars, 5.4 g fiber, 53 mg sodium

The Spicy One

MAKES 1 SERVING

1 large apple
2 stalks celery
1 cup chopped watercress
1 cup water
Juice of ½ lemon

Chop the apple, celery, and watercress. Add ingredients to blender and pulse until combined.

Per serving: 117 calories, 1.88 g protein, .54 g fat (.1 saturated), 29.61 g carbohydrates, 21.04 g sugars, 6 g fiber, 80 mg sodium

The Minty One

MAKES 1 SERVING

½ medium pear
¼ medium cucumber
½ cup chopped kale
½ cup chopped spinach
Juice of ½ lemon
5 peppermint leaves
1 cup ice cubes

Chop the pear and cucumber. Add the kale, spinach, lemon, and mint leaves to a blender and increase speed until the mixture is liquid. Add a quarter-cup of ice and blend, increasing ice by quarter-cup increments until the desired consistency is reached.

Per serving: 81 calories, 2.35 g protein, .54 g fat (.14 saturated), 19.83 g carbohydrates, 10.3 g sugars, 3.9 g fiber, 27 mg sodium

The Sweet One

MAKES 1 SERVING

½ medium banana, peeled
1 small orange, peeled
1 cup chopped kale
¼ cup water
1 cup ice cubes

Chop the banana and orange in half, and add to blender along with the kale and water. Blend until liquid. Add a quarter-cup of ice and blend, increasing ice by quarter-cup increments until the desired consistency is reached.

Per serving: 155 calories, 4.78 g protein, 1.02 g fat (.15 saturated), 36.90 g carbohydrates, 20.63 g sugars, 7 g fiber, 27 mg sodium

VEGETABLE-ONLY DINNERS

Lemon Pepper Vegetables

MAKES 1 SERVING

1 cup broccoli florets
1 cup snow peas, trimmed
1 cup sliced red bell pepper
Juice of ½ lemon
1 tablespoon olive oil
Freshly ground black pepper to taste

Place vegetables in a steamer basket or metal colander. Place inside a large pot filled with enough water to touch the bottom of the basket or colander. Bring water to a boil, placing lid on pot with a crack so that steam can escape, and cook vegetables for about 5 minutes or until they are tender. Remove from heat, place vegetables in a large bowl and drizzle with lemon juice, olive oil, and black pepper.

Squash and Greens

MAKES 1 SERVING

1 tablespoon coconut oil
2 cups kale, finely chopped
1 cup frozen butternut squash, defrosted
⅛ teaspoon nutmeg
¼ teaspoon cinnamon

Melt coconut oil in a medium sauté pan over medium heat. Sauté kale until wilted. Add butternut squash cubes and sauté until lightly browned, about 3–5 minutes. Add nutmeg and cinnamon; mix well and serve.

Rainbow Sauté

MAKES 1 SERVING

1 tablespoon olive oil
⅛ teaspoon red pepper flakes
⅛ teaspoon cumin
1½ cups cauliflower florets (cut small)
1 heaping cup chopped rainbow chard, finely chopped (include colorful stems)

In a medium sauté pan, heat olive oil over a low flame. Add red pepper flakes and cumin, shortly followed by cauliflower. Turn heat to medium and sauté for about 5–8 minutes or until tender. Add rainbow chard and sauté until wilted, 1–2 minutes. Place vegetables in a bowl and serve.

Asian Stir-Fry

1 tablespoon coconut oil
1 clove garlic, crushed and chopped
3 cups frozen Asian stir-fry mix (typical mixes include broccoli, snow peas, water chestnuts, red bell pepper)
½ teaspoon grated ginger

In a medium sauté pan, heat coconut oil over a low flame. Add garlic and sauté until fragrant. Add vegetables and turn heat up to medium-high, sautéing until soft, around 5 minutes. Add ginger and sauté for an additional minute. Place stir-fry in a large bowl and serve.

Dr. Taz's Kitchari

MAKES 4-6 SERVINGS

1 cup basmati rice, rinsed well

1 cup dry mung beans, soaked in water for 3 hours

4 cups water

2 teaspoons salt

1 teaspoon grated fresh ginger

1 tablespoon ghee or coconut oil

2 teaspoons turmeric

Mix ingredients in pressure cooker; keep under pressure for 6–7 minutes. If you don't have a pressure cooker, combine ingredients in a saucepan and bring to a boil. Reduce heat, cover, and simmer for approximately 45 minutes or until rice and mung beans are soft.

Dr. Taz's Sticky Rice

MAKES 4 SERVINGS

8 cups water

1 cup sticky or glutinous rice, rinsed well

½ teaspoon salt

4 quarter-inch slices of ginger

2 tablespoons olive oil or coconut oil

Bring water and rice to a boil. Reduce to simmer and add ginger and oil; cook for 30–40 minutes or until rice is ready to eat.

BONE BROTH SOUPS

Chicken Bone Broth Soup
MAKES 10–12 SERVINGS

2–3 pounds of bony chicken parts (wings, necks, etc.)
4 quarts cool, filtered water
2 tablespoons apple cider vinegar
3 carrots, peeled
2 medium onions, chopped
3 celery stalks chopped
¼ cup chopped parsley

Note: Farm-raised, free-range chickens give the best results.

Place the chicken pieces in a large pot with water, vinegar, and all vegetables except parsley. Let it sit for 30 minutes. Over medium flame, bring to a vigorous boil. Skim off any scum that rises to the top; reduce heat and cover. Simmer for a minimum of 8 hours. For more flavorful stock, simmer longer. Add the parsley for the final 15–30 minutes.

As the soup cools, use a slotted spoon to remove any large chicken and vegetable pieces. Strain out the remaining pieces through a metal colander and pour the broth into one large bowl or several small glass bowls. Chill in your refrigerator, skimming off any fat that congeals at the top. Store the broth in the refrigerator or freezer, depending on how quickly you plan to use it.

Slow Cooker Beef Bone Broth
MAKES 10–12 SERVINGS

1 medium carrot, chopped
1 medium celery rib, chopped
1 small onion, chopped
Around 2 pounds of beef bones

1 bay leaf

2 tablespoons apple cider vinegar

4 quarts cold, filtered water

Place the carrots, celery, onion, beef bones, bay leaf, vinegar, and water in the bottom of a 6-quart slow cooker. Make sure the ingredients are submerged; if not, add more water. Pour in enough water to submerge all of the ingredients. Set the slow cooker to low and set for a minimum of 8–10 hours and cover with lid (the longer you cook your soup, the more nutrients will be extracted from the bones). When the time is up, strain the ingredients so you are left with a translucent brown broth. Refrigerate broth overnight so you can scrape off and discard some of the solidified fat from the top. Reheat on stove when you are ready to eat it.

LEAN PROTEIN AND VEGETABLE DINNERS

Mexican Stir-Fry

MAKES 1 SERVING

2 teaspoons olive oil

Pinch of red pepper flakes

Pinch of cumin

4 ounces chicken breast, sliced

½ cup white button mushrooms, sliced

½ red bell pepper, sliced

½ green bell pepper, sliced

1 tablespoon chopped fresh cilantro

Heat oil in a medium saucepan. Add the red pepper flakes and cumin. Add chicken and sear for about one minute. Stir-fry for about 2 minutes, until mostly cooked. Add the remaining ingredients. Continue to stir-fry until the vegetables and chicken are fully cooked (about 5 minutes).

Herbed Turkey Breast and Sweet Potatoes

MAKES 1 SERVING

1 medium sweet potato

¼ teaspoon dried sage leaves

¼ teaspoon dried rosemary leaves

¼ teaspoon dried thyme leaves

1 4-ounce turkey breast cutlet

½ teaspoon olive oil

Preheat oven to 425°F. Scrub the sweet potato thoroughly with a brush under running water. Pat dry and poke with a fork. Wrap sweet potato in aluminum foil and bake for 45–60 minutes or until tender. Meanwhile, in a small dish, combine the sage, rosemary, and thyme leaves. Using your fingers, press the mixture onto the turkey breast. In a medium sauté pan or cast-iron skillet, heat one teaspoon of olive oil. Place the turkey cutlet in a hot pan and cook until bottom side is browned. Flip and brown on the other side, until cutlet is cooked through. Serve turkey and sweet potato together on plate, topping sweet potato with olive oil.

Spinach Sautéed in Olive Oil with Sole Topped with Lemon

MAKES 1 SERVING

1½ teaspoons olive oil (½ teaspoon + 1 teaspoon)

1 5-ounce sole fillet

3 cups baby spinach

½ lemon

Preheat oven to 400°F. Place sole in a shallow baking dish; drizzle both sides with a half-teaspoon of olive oil. Bake for about 30 minutes, or until fish is cooked through and beginning to flake, around 15 minutes (will vary depending on the thickness of the fish). While fish is cooking, pre-heat a medium sauté pan with the remaining teaspoon of olive oil. Add the garlic and spinach and sauté until the spinach is cooked. Place on dish next to the fish. Squeeze the half-lemon over it.

Ratatouille-Topped Chicken Breast

MAKES 1 SERVING

1½ teaspoons olive oil (1 teaspoon + ½ teaspoon)
½ small onion, diced
1 garlic clove, minced
½ cup eggplant, diced
3 or more tablespoons water
Pinch of salt
½ cup zucchini, diced
⅓ cup red bell pepper, diced
¾ cup tomatoes, chopped
1 tablespoon tomato paste
1 tablespoon basil, chopped
1 4-ounce chicken breast

Heat one teaspoon of olive oil in a medium sauté pan over a medium flame. Add the onions, cooking until translucent, about 5 minutes. Add the garlic and cook for another minute. Add the eggplant, two tablespoons of water, and salt and sauté until soft, adding additional water one table-spoon at a time as pan dries out; about 3–5 minutes. Add the zucchini and red bell pepper and cook for another 5 minutes. Add the tomato, basil, and tomato paste and mix, cooking for an additional 5 minutes.

While the vegetables are cooking, drizzle the chicken with the re-maining half-teaspoon oil and, using a grill pan or countertop grill, cook for around 5 minutes on either side or until cooked through. Place chicken breast on plate and top with ratatouille.

Note: To make this recipe vegetarian, eliminate the chicken, instead add-ing a half-cup of chickpeas when you add the tomatoes and basil.

Thanksgiving Dinner

MAKES 1 SERVING

1 small sweet potato
1½ cups sliced Brussels sprouts
2 teaspoons coconut oil (1 teaspoon + 1 teaspoon)
1 4-ounce turkey breast cutlet

Preheat oven to 425°F. Scrub the sweet potato thoroughly with a brush under running water. With a fork, poke holes in the sweet potato and wrap in aluminum foil. Bake until tender, about 45–60 minutes. At the same time, place Brussels sprouts in a cast-iron pan or on a baking tray and toss with one teaspoon of coconut oil. Bake for about 25–30 minutes or until Brussels sprouts become browned, tossing every 10 minutes. In the meantime, heat a small skillet with the rest of the coconut oil. Cook the turkey breast cutlet on one side until browned, flip, and cook on other side until cooked through. Serve turkey, sweet potato, and Brussels sprouts together on a plate.

Steamed Artichoke with Baked Flounder

MAKES 1 SERVING

1 medium artichoke
1 5–6-ounce flounder fillet
2 teaspoons olive oil
Pinch of dried oregano

Preheat oven to 425°F. In a small pot, add water up about one inch and bring to a boil. Trim off the top inch of the artichoke and pull off any small leaves around the base. Place artichoke in water, bottom side up, and simmer with the lid on for about 20–30 minutes or until you can easily insert a fork into the base. While artichoke is simmering, place flounder in a shallow baking dish, drizzled with a half-teaspoon of olive oil. Bake until fish can be easily flaked with a fork and is cooked through, around

8 minutes (will vary depending on thickness). In a small bowl, sprinkle remaining olive oil with oregano as a dipping sauce for the artichoke. Drain artichoke and serve along with the flounder.

Baked Spaghetti Squash with
Tomato Sauce and Chicken Breast

MAKES 1 SERVING

1 small spaghetti squash
1 4-ounce chicken breast
1 teaspoon olive oil
1 clove of garlic, crushed
½ cup canned tomatoes, diced
⅛ teaspoon oregano

Preheat oven to 375°F. Cut a small slice off one end of the squash length-wise so you can rest it on a baking dish and poke holes in the top with a fork. Place the squash in the baking dish and roast for about 45 minutes or until a fork can easily puncture the skin. Using a grill pan or countertop grill, cook the chicken breast until cooked through, about 5 minutes on each side. While the chicken breast is cooking, heat the olive oil in a small pan over medium heat. Add the garlic, tomatoes, and oregano and cook for about 5 minutes. When the spaghetti squash is ready, remove strands from the skin, place in a large bowl, and top with the tomato mixture and grilled chicken breast.

Turkey with Braised Root Vegetables

MAKES 1 SERVING

2 large carrots
1 large parsnip
1 small celery root
1½ teaspoons olive oil (1 teaspoon + ½ teaspoon)
½ cup water

½ teaspoon chopped fresh parsley

1 4-ounce turkey breast

Scrub the carrots, parsnips, and celery root and chop into bite-size pieces. Heat 1 teaspoon of oil in a sauté pan over medium flame. Add vegetables and sauté for about 5 minutes or until lightly browned. Add water and bring to a boil. Reduce to a simmer, cover pan, and cook until vegetables soften (around 15–20 minutes), removing the lid and adding parsley for the last minute or so. As vegetables are cooking, heat a small skillet with the rest of the olive oil. Cook the turkey breast on one side until browned, flip, and cook on other side until cooked through. Serve turkey and root vegetables together on plate.

Broiled Ginger Halibut with Mashed Turnips

MAKES 1 SERVING

2 cups turnips, diced into 1-inch cubes

1 5-ounce halibut fillet

1 clove garlic, chopped

¼ teaspoon grated fresh ginger

½ teaspoon olive oil

½ teaspoon coconut oil

1 teaspoon chopped cilantro

Bring a medium pot of water to a boil over a high heat. Add turnips and cook until tender, 20–30 minutes. In the meantime, line a broiler pan with foil and preheat in broiler for 5 minutes. Remove the pan from the oven and place the fish in the center, sprinkling with garlic, ginger, and olive oil. Return to broiler and cook until fish is just cooked through, around 8–10 minutes. Place on serving plate. When turnips are fork-tender, re-move from heat and drain water thoroughly. Return turnips to pot and add the coconut oil and cilantro. Blend using a potato masher until rela-tively smooth. Serve on plate beside halibut.

Mexican Veggie Bowl
MAKES 1 SERVING

1 teaspoon olive oil
½ cup chopped zucchini
½ cup chopped carrots
½ cup black beans, rinsed and drained
¼ cup prepared salsa
¼ lime

In a small sauté pan, preheat olive oil over a medium flame. Add the zucchini and carrots and sauté until softened, about 5–7 minutes. Drain off any remaining liquid. Place in a large bowl and top with black beans and salsa; squeeze with lime.

PROBIOTIC FOODS

Sauerkraut
MAKES 6-8 SERVINGS

1 medium head of green or red cabbage
1½ tablespoons sea or kosher salt

Supplies: Cutting board, large knife, large mixing bowl, large mason jar, cheesecloth, rubber band, fork.

Give all of your supplies (including your hands) a good cleaning—you want the bacteria on the surface of the cabbage to not have to compete with any other microbes. Remove the limp outer leaves of the cabbage and set aside. Chop the cabbage, removing the tough inner core, and shred the rest. Transfer to the bowl and sprinkle with salt. Massage the salt into the shredded cabbage using your hands until the cabbage becomes watery. Using your hands, pack the cabbage into the mason jar. Pour the remaining liquid on top of the shredded cabbage. Use one of the outer leaves of the cabbage to weigh down the shredded cabbage to ensure that it stays submerged in its liquid. Cover the mouth of the jar with cheesecloth and secure with a rubber band. Every few hours, remove the cheesecloth and press the cabbage down with a fork so that it is even more submerged in the liquid. Return cheesecloth and allow to ferment in a cool, dark place for three or more days. Once you like the flavor of the sauerkraut, replace the cheesecloth with a lid and store it in the refrigerator for up to two months.

Kimchi

MAKES 6-8 SERVINGS

1 Napa cabbage (around 2 pounds)
¼ cup sea or kosher salt
1 teaspoon sugar
2 teaspoons grated ginger
1 tablespoon minced garlic (about 6 cloves)
3–4 tablespoons spring water or filtered water
1–5 tablespoons Korean red pepper flakes, also called kochugaru, depending on your desire/tolerance for heat
4 scallions, trimmed and cut into 1-inch pieces
8 ounces daikon, peeled and cut into matchsticks

Clean your hands and supplies well. Cut the cabbage into four equal quarters and remove the tough inner core. Cut each quarter across, into 2-inch-wide strips. Place the cabbage in a large bowl and sprinkle with salt. Use your hands to massage the salt into the cabbage until it begins to turn soft. Submerge the cabbage in the spring or filtered water and let stand for 1–2 hours, turning it once halfway through. Rinse the cabbage well under cold water three times. Pour it into a colander and drain it for 15–30 minutes. In the meantime, clean the bowl you used for salting and set it aside for later. In a small bowl, combine the sugar, ginger, garlic,

3 to 4 tablespoons of spring or filtered water, and the Korean red pepper flakes and mix to form a smooth paste. Squeeze any excess water from the cabbage and put it back into the large bowl. Add the scallions, daikon, and paste to the bowl, mixing everything together until the vegetables are evenly mixed and thoroughly coated with the paste (use your hands—gloves optional). Pack the kimchi into a large glass jar with a tight-fitting lid, pushing the cabbage down so that brine covers the vegetables. Leaving one inch empty at the top, seal the jar with the lid. Let the jar stand at room temperature for 5–14 days on a plate or in a bowl, since some of the brine can seep out of the jar. Check on the kimchi once a day, pressing down on the vegetables to ensure that they remain submerged in brine. Refrigerate before eating and keep for up to a month.

Ginger Miso Stir-Fry Sauce

MAKES 4-6 SERVINGS

½ cup hot water
¼ cup white miso
1 tablespoon toasted sesame oil
2 teaspoons grated fresh ginger
1 clove garlic, crushed and minced

Whisk the ingredients together in a small bowl. Add to stir-fried vegetables for the last 1–2 minutes of cooking.

Coconut Miso Stir-Fry Sauce

MAKES 4-6 SERVINGS

¼ cup white miso
¼ cup hot water
½ cup canned coconut milk
3 tablespoons chopped cilantro

Dissolve miso in hot water. Whisk in coconut milk and add cilantro. Add to stir-fried vegetables for the last 1–2 minutes of cooking.

Lemony Miso Tahini Dressing
MAKES 4-6 SERVINGS

¼ cup white miso
¼ cup tahini
Juice of ½ lemon
Hot water

Whisk together ingredients, adding water until the desired consistency is achieved. Use to dress steamed vegetables or as a dipping sauce for vegetables (you might want to leave it a bit thicker for this purpose).

Tempeh Dipping Sticks
MAKES 2 SERVINGS

1 block tempeh
2 tablespoons coconut oil

Preheat oven to 375°F. Slice block of tempeh into finger-length strips about a quarter-inch thick. Grease a cast-iron pan or baking sheet with one tablespoon of coconut oil. Arrange tempeh neatly and bake for about 15–20 minutes or until the bottom side begins to form a crust. Flip pieces with a spatula, add the other tablespoon of coconut oil, and cook another 15–20 minutes or until browned on both sides.

PREBIOTIC FOODS

Baked Jerusalem Artichokes
MAKES 4-6 SERVINGS

2 pounds Jerusalem artichokes
2 teaspoons olive oil

Preheat oven to 375°F. Scrub Jerusalem artichokes and cut into one-inch cubes. Spread onto baking sheet and drizzle with olive oil, tossing to distribute. Roast for about 45 minutes or until golden brown, tossing every 5–10 minutes.

Miso Bowl
MAKES 1 SERVING

½ teaspoon olive oil
4 cups baby arugula
1 4-ounce chicken breast
¼ cup sliced red onion
¼ avocado
2 tablespoons ginger miso sauce or lemony miso tahini dressing

In a medium skillet over a medium flame, heat olive oil. Add arugula and sauté until wilted. Place in a medium bowl. In the same pan, cook chicken breast for about 5 minutes on each side, until cooked through. Place in the bowl on top of the arugula and top with the red onion, avocado, and miso dressing of your choice.

ADDITIONAL RECIPES

Beef and Pepper Stir-Fry

MAKES 1 SERVING

1 teaspoon olive oil

4 ounces lean beef, sliced thinly (no more than a half-inch thick)

½ red bell pepper, sliced

½ green bell pepper, sliced

In a medium skillet over a medium flame, heat olive oil. Add beef slices—meat should sizzle when it hits the pan. Cook 2–3 minutes per side, or until cooked through. Add red and green bell pepper and sauté for about one minute. Place mixture in a large bowl and serve.

Tempeh Reuben

MAKES 1 SERVING

1 teaspoon olive oil

3 ounces grilled tempeh, sliced thinly

1 slice Swiss cheese

2 slices sprouted grain bread

¼ cup sauerkraut

⅛ avocado, sliced

1 teaspoon Russian dressing

In a small skillet, heat oil over a medium-high flame. Cook tempeh slices for 2 minutes each side, until lightly browned, about 2–3 minutes on each side. Remove from skillet and add both slices of bread to the skillet. Place cheese on one slice of bread and toast until melted. Remove bread slices from skillet and stack tempeh, sauerkraut, avocado and dressing on top of the cheese. Place the other slice of bread on top and serve.

Quinoa-Stuffed Squash with Lemon Sole

MAKES 1 SERVING

Squash

½ butternut squash, cleaned and seeds removed

1 teaspoon coconut oil

½ cup baby spinach

½ cup cooked quinoa

Sole

1 5-ounce sole fillet

½ teaspoon olive oil

¼ lemon

Preheat oven to 400°F. Place butternut squash facedown on a baking sheet and cook until flesh is soft, about 40 minutes. On another baking sheet, place sole on a sheet of aluminum foil, drizzle with oil, and tent the top. Bake until cooked through, 6–12 minutes depending on the thickness of the fish. In the meantime, in a medium skillet over medium heat, cook baby spinach in coconut oil until wilted. Add quinoa and mix well. When squash is finished, fill empty cavity with spinach quinoa mixture. Serve with sole, drizzled with juice from the lemon.

Green Egg Scramble

MAKES 1 SERVING

1 teaspoon olive oil

½ cup white button mushrooms, sliced

2 cups baby spinach

1–2 large eggs

¼ avocado

In a medium skillet, heat oil over a medium flame. Add mushrooms and cook until soft, about 2 minutes. Add spinach and cook until wilted. In a small bowl, whisk egg or eggs. Add to skillet, stirring gently so that the egg and vegetables form a uniform mixture. Cook, gently scrambling, until egg sets. Pour the egg and vegetable scramble onto plate and top with avocado.

Greek Chicken
MAKES 1 SERVING

1 teaspoon olive oil
4 ounces chicken breast
⅓ cup chopped red onion
⅓ cup chopped green pepper
⅓ cup chopped tomato
1 ounce feta cheese

Heat oil in a small skillet over medium heat. Cook chicken until cooked through, about 5 minutes on each side. Place chicken on a dish; in the same skillet, sauté onions until soft. Add green pepper and cook for another 1–2 minutes; add tomato and cook for another minute, scraping up browned pieces from bottom of pan. Pour mixture on top of chicken and top with feta cheese.

CHAPTER 10/DIET MODIFICATION RECIPES

Chopped Garlic and Herb Dressing
MAKES 4 SERVINGS

¼ cup olive oil
1 tablespoon lemon juice
2 garlic cloves, minced
1 tablespoon minced fresh thyme
Salt and pepper to taste

In a small bowl, whisk the olive oil and lemon juice together until well blended. Mix in the garlic and thyme until combined. Use to dress cooked meat, vegetables, and more.

Vegetarian Miso Soup

MAKES 4 SERVINGS

4 cups water
1 sheet nori (dried seaweed)
4 tablespoons white miso paste
1 cup spinach, finely chopped

In a medium pot, bring the water to a boil. Cut nori into eight pieces lengthwise and drop in water, reducing heat to a simmer. Cook for about 5 minutes. While the nori is cooking, place the miso paste in a small bowl and whisk with a bit of hot water, smoothing out any lumps. Add miso to the pot of simmering water and mix well. Add spinach and cook for an additional 5 minutes.

Notes

INTRODUCTION

xiii   **"Bacteria in the Intestines"**   Denise Grady, "Bacteria in the Intestines May Help Tip the Bathroom Scale, Studies Show," *New York Times,* March 7, 2013, accessed May 9, 2014, available at www.nytimes.com/2013/03/28/health/studies-focus-on-gut-bacteria-in-weight -loss.html.

xiii   **"The Humble Heroes"**   Virginia Hughes, "The Humble Heroes of Weight-Loss Surgery: Stomach Acids and Gut Microbes," *National Geographic,* March 2013, accessed May 9, 2014, available at http://phenomena.nationalgeographic.com/2014/03/26/the -humble-heroes-of-weight-loss-surgery-stomach-acids-and-gut-microbes/.

xiii   **"wellbeing in innumerable ways"**   Wendy Garrett, "Bacterial Metabolites Regulate Immune System Function in the Colon and May Help Reduce Inflammatory Bowel Disease," *Harvard School of Public Health News,* July 29, 2013, accessed May 9, 2014, available at www .hsph.harvard.edu/news/features/bacterial-metabolites-regulate-immune-system-function -in-the-colon-and-may-help-reduce-inflammatory-bowel-disease/.

xiv   **may be able to reverse it**   Kanakaraju Kaliannan et al., "Intestinal Alkaline Phosphatase Prevents Metabolic Syndrome in Mice," accessed May 10, 2014, available at www.pnas.org /content/early/2013/04/04/1220180110.

xiv   **gut bacteria into sterile mice**   Garrett, "Bacterial Metabolites Regulate Immune System Function."

xv   **recent study in *Proceedings of the National Academy of Sciences***   Javier A. Bravo et al., "Ingestion of *Lactobacillus* Strain Regulates Emotional Behavior and Central GABA Receptor Expression in a Mouse via the Vagus Nerve," *Proceedings of the National Academy of Sciences,* accessed May 10, 2014, available at www.pnas.org/content/early/2011/08/26 /1102999108.

xvi   **aren't even supposed to touch it**   "Finasteride," MedLinePlus, last modified January 15, 2012, accessed April 13, 2014, available at www.nlm.nih.gov/medlineplus/druginfo/meds /a698016.html.

xvi   **Chinese medicine was teaching**   "Digestive Health = Total Body Health," September 28,

2011, updated January 30, 2014, American College for Advancement in Medicine website, accessed April 13, 2014, available at www.acam.org/blogpost/1092863/180732/Digestive-Health--Total-Body-Health.

xix **gluten intolerance and celiac disease** M. de Lorgeril and P. Salen, "Gluten and Wheat Intolerance Today: Are Modern Wheat Strains Involved?" *International Journal of Food Sciences and Nutrition,* published online February 13, 2014, accessed April 14, 2014, available at www.ncbi.nlm.nih.gov/pubmed/24524657.

xx **a vegetarian diet, and regular exercise** John Harvey Kellogg Papers, Bentley Historical Library, University of Michigan, accessed April 13, 2014, available at http://quod.lib.umich.edu/b/bhlead/umich-bhl-851724?rgn=main;view=text.

xx **it must be said, went too far** Dale Keiger, "The 'Good Conduct' of Sex," *John Hopkins Magazine,* June 2000, accessed April 13, 2014, available at www.jhu.edu/jhumag/0600web/arts.html#sex.

xxi **contributing to chronic illness** Lawrence A. David et al., "Diet Rapidly and Reproducibly Alters the Human Gut Microbiome," *Nature* 505 (January 23, 2014): 559–63, doi:10.1038/nature12820, published online December 11, 2013, accessed April 13, 2014, available at www.nature.com/nature/journal/vaop/ncurrent/full/nature12820.html.

xxi **your tendency to gain weight** Emmanuelle Le Chatelier et al., "Richness of Human Gut Microbiome Correlates with Metabolic Markers," *Nature* 500, no. 7464 (August 29, 2013): 541–46, doi:10.1038/nature12506, accessed April 15, 2014, available at www.nature.com/nature/journal/v500/n7464/full/nature12506.html.

xxi **associated with anxiety or depression** Suzanne Morrison, "That Anxiety May Be in Your Gut, Not Your Head," McMaster University news release, published May 17, 2011, accessed April 13, 2014, available at http://fhs.mcmaster.ca/main/news/news_2011/gut_anxiety_link_study.html.

xxi **abnormal bacterial content in the gut** Morrison, "That Anxiety May Be in Your Gut."

xxi **perhaps other autoimmune diseases** Carol Torgan, "Gut Microbes Linked to Rheumatoid Arthritis," *NIH Research Matters,* National Institutes of Health website, published November 25, 2013, accessed April 13, 2014, available at www.nih.gov/researchmatters/november2013/11252013arthritis.htm.

xxi **role against this chronic disease** J. Qin et al., "A Metagenome-Wide Association Study of Gut Microbiota in Type 2 Diabetes," *Nature* 490, no. 7418 (October 4, 2012): 55–60, doi:10.1038/nature11450, accessed April 13, 2014, available at www.ncbi.nlm.nih.gov/pubmed/23023125.

xxii **gas pills, antacids, and the like** "Digestive Health = Total Body Health."

xxii **up to 20 percent of Americans** Digestive Diseases Statistics for the United States, U.S. Department of Health and Human Services, National Digestive Diseases. Information Clearinghouse (NDDIC), Page last updated September 10, 2013, accessed April 13, 2014, available at http://digestive.niddk.nih.gov/statistics/statistics.aspx#1.

xxiii **you're likely familiar with: obesity** E. Ness-Jensen et al., "Changes in Prevalence, Incidence and Spontaneous Loss of Gastro-Oesophageal Reflux Symptoms: A Prospective Population-Based Cohort Study, the HUNT Study," *Gut* 61, no. 10 (October 2012): 1390–97, doi:10.1136/gutjnl-2011-300715, accessed April 13, 2014, available at www.ncbi.nlm.nih.gov/pubmed?term=22190483.

CHAPTER 1. THE FIRE IN YOUR BELLY

3 **as unique as your fingerprint** "Everything You Always Wanted to Know About the Gut Microbiota . . ." Gut Microbiota Worldwatch, public information service from European Society of Neurogastroenterology and Motility, accessed April 14, 2014, available at www.gutmicrobiotawatch.org/gut-microbiota-info/.

3 **gut bugs coexist peacefully** "NIH Human Microbiome Project Defines Normal Bacterial

Makeup of the Body," news release, National Institutes of Health, published June 13, 2012, accessed April 14, 2014, available at www.nih.gov/news/health/jun2012/nhgri-13.htm.

3   **But too many of the wrong**   "Everything You Always Wanted to Know About the Gut Microbiota . . ."

6   **fluid around the injured area**   Cynthia Johnson and Pamela Jones, "Chronic Inflammation and Disease," NYU Langone Medical Center website, last reviewed November 2013, accessed April 15, 2014, available at www.med.nyu.edu/content?ChunkIID=882153.

6   **food particles your gut can't digest**   E. Shacter and S. A. Weitzman, "Chronic Inflammation and Cancer," *Oncology* 16, no. 2 (February 2002): 217–26, 229; discussion 230–32, accessed April 14, 2014, available at www.ncbi.nlm.nih.gov/pubmed/11866137.

6   **the two most common types of inflammatory bowel disease**   "Inflammatory Bowel Disease," National Centers for Disease Control website, last updated January 14, 2014, accessed April 14, 2014, available at www.cdc.gov/ibd/.

6   **Both gut dysbiosis and a leaky gut**   M. F. Gregor and G. S. Hotamisligil, "Inflammatory Mechanisms in Obesity," *Annual Review of Immunology* 29 (2011):415–45, doi:10.1146/annurev-immunol-031210-101322, accessed April 14, 2014, available at www.ncbi.nlm.nih.gov/pubmed/21219177.

8   **is the science of life**   "Ayurvedic Medicine: An Introduction," National Center for Complementary and Alternative Medicine website, updated August 2013, accessed April 14, 2014, available at http://nccam.nih.gov/health/ayurveda/introduction.htm.

8   **earth, air, fire, water, and space**   "What Is the Philosophy of Ayurvedic Medicine?" University of Minnesota website, accessed April 14, 2014, available at www.takingcharge.csh.umn.edu/explore-healing-practices/ayurvedic-medicine/what-philosophy-ayurvedic-medicine.

8   **while earth is solid and stable**   "Ayurveda Certificate Programs," Southern California University of Health Sciences website, accessed April 14, 2014, available at www.scuhs.edu/academics/sps/ayurveda/.

8   **are typically aggressive achievers**   "What Is the Philosophy of Ayurvedic Medicine?"

8   **diarrhea, rashes, and anger**   Ibid.

9   **typically quick, alert, and restless**   Ibid.

9   **to fuel creativity and clear comprehension**   Ibid.

9   **get frequent exercise, and avoid naps**   Ibid.

10   **disease for over 2,500 years**   "Traditional Chinese Medicine: An Introduction," National Center for Complementary and Alternative Medicine website, updated October 2013, accessed April 14, 2014, available at http://nccam.nih.gov/health/whatiscam/chinesemed.htm.

10   **yin and yang must be maintained or restored**   "Theory and Practice for Traditional Chinese Medicine," Pacific College of Oriental Medicine website, accessed April 14, 2014, available at www.pacificcollege.edu/acupuncture-massage-news/articles/471-theory-and-practice-for-traditional-chinese-medicine.html#sthash.IrdZDIQZ.9b03B4Lf.dpuf.

11   **"cold" and "hot" foods for you**   Ibid.

11   **liquid extracts, and powders**   "Traditional Chinese Medicine: An Introduction."

11   **metal needles at these points releases qi**   Ibid.

12   **breathing and relaxation**   Ibid.

12   **The United States accredits schools in Chinese medicine**   "Acupuncture and Traditional Chinese Medicine Schools," Acupuncture Today website, accessed April 14, 2014, available at www.acupuncturetoday.com/abc/acupuncture_schools.php.

15   **tenfold increased risk for the disease**   Yuri A. Saito, "The Role of Genetics in IBS," *Gastroenterology Clinics of North America* 40, no. 1 (March 2011): 45–67, doi:10.1016/j.gtc.2010.12.011, accessed April 14, 2014, available at www.ncbi.nlm.nih.gov/pmc/articles/PMC3056499/.

15   **become incorporated into the gut**   "Gut Microbes and Diet Interact to Affect Obesity," NIH Research Matters website, National Institutes of Health, published September 16,

2013, accessed April 14, 2014, available at www.nih.gov/researchmatters/september2013/09162013obesity.htm.

CHAPTER 2. THE "GUTS" OF YOUR GUT

19   **can undermine its ability to recover**   Woods Hole Center for Oceans and Human Health website, accessed April 14, 2014, available at www.whoi.edu/whcohh/.

19   **just under the surface of the gut lining**   Kathleen Wong, "Gut Feeling," *Breakthroughs,* College of Natural Resources, University of California at Berkeley, fall 2007, accessed April 14, 2014, available at http://nature.berkeley.edu/breakthroughs/break_feature2_fa07.php.

20   **in the ability of the blood to clot**   "Vitamin K," MedLinePlus, reviewed October 23, 2012, accessed April 13, 2014, available at www.nlm.nih.gov/medlineplus/druginfo/natural/983.html.

20   **the liver, pancreas, and gallbladder**   "The Digestive System and How It Works," National Digestive Diseases Information Clearinghouse, NIH Publication 13-2681, updated September 18, 2013, accessed April 14, 2014, available at http://digestive.niddk.nih.gov/ddiseases/pubs/yrdd/.

21   **and soul-satisfying elimination**   Ibid.

21   **blood flow to your digestive organs**   S. A. Giduck et al., "Cephalic Reflexes: Their Role in Digestion and Possible Roles in Absorption and Metabolism," *Journal of Nutrition* 117, no. 7 (July 1987): 1191–96, accessed April 14, 2014, available at http://jn.nutrition.org/content/117/7/1191.long.

23   **it's called peristalsis**   "Normal Gastrointestinal Motility and Function," University of North Carolina Center for Functional GI and Motility Disorders, accessed April 14, 2014, available at www.med.unc.edu/ibs/files/educational-gi-handouts/GI%20Motility%20Functions.pdf.

23   **and back into the esophagus**   "Gastroesophageal Reflux Disease," MedLinePlus, modified August 11, 2011, accessed April 14, 2014, available at www.nlm.nih.gov/medlineplus/ency/article/000265.htm.

23   **reflux, or gastroesophageal reflux**   "Esophagus Disorders," MedLinePlus, accessed April 14, 2014, available at www.nlm.nih.gov/medlineplus/esophagusdisorders.html.

24   **That's as strong as battery acid!**   "Strength of Acids," Argonne National Laboratory website, accessed April 14, 2014, available at www.newton.dep.anl.gov/askasci/chem00/chem00998.htm.

25   **moment food from the esophagus hits it**   "The Digestive System and How It Works."

26   **migraines to hypothyroidism, IBS, and fibromyalgia**   "Association Between Hypothyroidism and Small Intestinal Bacterial Overgrowth," JCEM 2007, available at http://press.endocrine.org/doi/full/10.1210/jc.2007-0606; "A Link Between Irritable Bowel Syndrome and Fibromyalgia May Be Related to Findings on Lactulose Breath Testing," ARD 2004, available at http://ard.bmj.com/content/63⁄4/450.full.

27   **allergic reaction of anaphylaxis can occur**   James Li, "What's the Difference Between a Food Intolerance and Food Allergy?" accessed April 14, 2014, available at www.mayoclinic.org/diseases-conditions/food-allergy/expert-answers/food-allergy/FAQ-20058538?p=1.

27   **peanuts, tree nuts, soy, and wheat**   "Food Allergy," MedLinePlus, accessed April 14, 2014, available at www.nlm.nih.gov/medlineplus/foodallergy.html.

27   **not life-threatening, as a food allergy can be**   Li, "What's the Difference Between a Food Intolerance and Food Allergy?"

28   **liquefied meal into your small intestine**   "Your Gastrointestinal System: What It Is and How It Works," NYU Langone Medical Center website, accessed April 14, 2014, available at http://medicine.med.nyu.edu/gastro/digestive-health/your-digestive-health#sthash.0B02vPVm.dpuf.

28   **2.5 gallons of food, liquids, and waste a day**   "Small Intestine," innerbody.com, accessed April 14, 2014, available at www.innerbody.com/image_digeov/dige10-new3.html.

28   **It's these tiny, hairlike projections**   Ibid.

28   **The other symptoms of CD**   "Celiac Disease," National Digestive Diseases Information Clearinghouse, NIH Publication 13-2681, updated January 27, 2012, accessed April 14, 2014, available at http://digestive.niddk.nih.gov/ddiseases/pubs/celiac/.

30   **Leaky gut may be the culprit**   "What Is Celiac Disease?" Celiac Disease Foundation website, accessed April 14, 2014, available at http://celiac.org/celiac-disease/what-is-celiac-disease/.

30   **so that the body can eliminate it**   "Your Gastrointestinal System: What It Is and How It Works," NYU Langone Medical Center website, accessed April 14, 2014, available at http://medicine.med.nyu.edu/gastro/digestive-health/your-digestive-health#sthash.0B02v PVm.dpuf.

36   **functions well, breaking down fats**   "How Does the Liver Work?" PubMed Health, updated November 22, 2012, accessed April 14, 2014, available at www.ncbi.nlm.nih.gov /pubmedhealth/PMH0015941/.

36   **environmental chemicals from your blood**   "Facts About the Liver," Children's Hospital of Philadelphia website, October 2012, accessed April 14, 2014, available at www.chop .edu/service/liver-transplant-program/about-liver-transplant/liver-anatomy-and-function .html.

37   **it now increasingly affects children**   "Fatty Liver Disease," Weight-Control Information Network website, a division of National Institute of Diabetes and Digestive and Kidney Diseases, accessed April 14, 2014, available at http://win.niddk.nih.gov/publications/health _risks.htm#i.

38   **The enzymes this organ makes**   "The Pancreas," Sol Goldman Pancreatic Cancer Research Center at Johns Hopkins website, accessed April 14, 2014, available at http:// pathology.jhu.edu/pancreas/BasicOverview1.php?area=ba.

38   **sugar, called glucose, for energy**   Ibid.

38   **can lead to prediabetes or type 2 diabetes**   "Insulin Resistance and Prediabetes," National Diabetes Information Clearinghouse website, NIH Publication 13-4893, updated January 22, 2013, accessed April 14, 2014, available at http://diabetes.niddk.nih.gov/dm/pubs /insulinresistance/.

38   **increases the risk of a heart attack or stroke**   "Heart Disease," American Diabetes Association website, accessed April 14, 2014, available at www.diabetes.org/living-with-diabetes /complications/heart-disease/.

CHAPTER 3. THE BRAIN IN YOUR BELLY

40   **in its sophistication and complexity**   "Neurogastroenterology," Clinical Summary, updated July 22, 2013, accessed April 15, 2014, available at www.medlink.com/medlinkcontent.asp.

40   **Scientists have just begun to**   Michael D. Gershon, *The Second Brain: A Groundbreaking New Understanding of Nervous Disorders of the Stomach and Intestine* (New York: Harper, 1998, republished 2003), xiii–xiv.

40   **anxiety, stress, or depression—or a reaction to it**   Peera Hemarajata and James Versalovic, "Effects of Probiotics on Gut Microbiota: Mechanisms of Intestinal Immunomodulation and Neuromodulation," *Therapeutic Advances in Gastroenterology* 6, no. 1 (January 2013): 39–51, doi:10.1177/1756283X12459294, accessed April 15, 2014, available at www .ncbi.nlm.nih.gov/pmc/articles/PMC3539293/.

41   **to each other and to the cells they control**   Gershon, *Second Brain,* xiii.

43   **building blocks of the brain and nervous system**   "Brain Basics," National Institute of Mental Health website, accessed April 15, 2014, available at www.nimh.nih.gov/health /educational-resources/brain-basics/brain-basics.shtml.

43   **more than are in your spine**   Tim Taylor, "Nervous System," innerbody.com, accessed April 15, 2014, available at www.innerbody.com/image/nervov.html.

43   **sleep, and digestion, among other processes**   Adam Hadhazy, "Think Twice: How the Gut's 'Second Brain' Influences Mood and Well Being," *Scientific American,* published February 12, 2010, accessed April 15, 2014, available at www.scientificamerican.com /article/gut-second-brain/.

43   **between neurons called synapses**   "Brain Basics."

43   **and ends in your belly**   "Vagus Nerve Stimulation," NYU Langone Medical Center website, accessed April 15, 2014, available at http://epilepsy.med.nyu.edu/diagnosis-treatment /vagus-nerve-stimulation-vns#sthash.V0EJZiSY.HNz2F9ne.dpbs.

43   **that keeps the gut and brain "connected"**   Rob Stein, "Gut Bacteria Might Guide the Workings of Our Minds," National Public Radio website, published November 18, 2013, accessed April 15, 2014, available at www.npr.org/blogs/health/2013/11/18/244526773/gut -bacteria-might-guide-the-workings-of-our-minds.

44   **induce our adrenal glands**   "Catecholamines—Blood," MedLinePlus, last modified January 26, 2013, accessed April 15, 2014, available at www.nlm.nih.gov/medlineplus/ency /article/003561.htm.

44   **in the fight-or-flight response**   "Cortisol Level," MedLinePlus, last modified December 11, 2011, accessed April 15, 2014, available at www.nlm.nih.gov/medlineplus/ency /article/003693.htm.

45   **get out of bed in the morning**   Alex Kecskes, "Traditional Chinese Medicine Can Help Adrenal Fatigue," Pacific College of Oriental Medicine website, accessed April 15, 2014, available at www.pacificcollege.edu/acupuncture-massage-news/articles/745-traditional -chinese-medicine-can-help-adrenal-fatigue.html.

45   **"the hunger hormone"**   Anne Trafton, "New Role for 'Hunger Hormone,'" news release, Massachusetts Institute of Technology website, October 15, 2013, accessed April 15, 2014, available at http://newsoffice.mit.edu/2013/ghrelin-ptsd-1015.

46   **serotonin promotes restful sleep**   "Tryptophan," MedLinePlus, last modified February 7, 2010, accessed April 15, 2014, available at www.nlm.nih.gov/medlineplus/ency/article /002332.htm.

46   **determines whether serotonin is broken down**   Marcus Manocha and Waliul I. Khan, "Serotonin and GI Disorders: An Update on Clinical and Experimental Studies," *Clinical and Translational Gastroenterology* (2012): 3, e13; doi:10.1038/ctg.2012.8, published online April 26, 2012, accessed April 15, 2014, available at www.nature.com/ctg/journal/v3/n4 /full/ctg20128a.html.

46   **to sensations like fullness or pain**   Christine Case-Lo, "IBS and Serotonin: The Brain and Stomach Link," Healthline website, accessed April 15, 2014, available at www.healthline .com/health/irritable-bowel-syndrome/serotonin-effects.

46   **serotonin levels are a significant factor in IBS**   Manocha and Khan, "Serotonin and GI Disorders."

47   **another 18 percent anxiety disorders**   "The Numbers Count: Mental Disorders in America," National Institute of Mental Health website, accessed April 15, 2014, available at www.nimh.nih.gov/health/publications/the-numbers-count-mental-disorders-in-america /index.shtml#MajorDepressive.

47   **biological, environmental, and psychological factors**   "What Is Depression?" National Institute of Mental Health website, NIH Publication 11-3561, revised 2011, accessed April 15, 2014, available at www.nimh.nih.gov/health/publications/depression/index .shtml#pub5; "What Is Anxiety Disorder?" National Institute of Mental Health website, accessed April 15, 2014, available at www.nimh.nih.gov/health/topics/anxiety-disorders /index.shtml#part2.

47   **depression can improve gut issues**   Siri Carpenter, "That Gut Feeling," American Psychology Association, *Monitor on Psychology* 43, no. 8 (September 2012): 50, accessed April 15, 2014, available at www.apa.org/monitor/2012/09/gut-feeling.aspx.

47 **suffer from anxiety and depression** Ibid.

48 **the pathology of depression, the study found** M. Maes et al., "The Gut-Brain Barrier in Major Depression: Intestinal Mucosal Dysfunction with an Increased Translocation of LPS from Gram Negative Enterobacteria (Leaky Gut) Plays a Role in the Inflammatory Pathophysiology of Depression," *Neuroendocrinology Letters* 29, no. 1 (February 2008): 117–24, accessed April 15, 2014, available at www.ncbi.nlm.nih.gov/pubmed/18283240.

48 **(such as tartrazine, benzoates, and sorbates)** Yurdagül Zopf et al., "The Differential Diagnosis of Food Intolerance," *Deutsches Ärzteblatt International* 106, no. 21 (May 2009): 359–70, 2009. doi:10.3238/arztebl.2009.0359, published online May 22, 2009, accessed April 15, 2014, available at www.ncbi.nlm.nih.gov/pmc/articles/PMC2695393/.

49 **wood type typically exhibits more aggression** Eric L. Goldman, "The Five Faces of ADHD: A Chinese Medicine Approach," *Holistic Primary Care* 8, no. 2 (Summer 2007), accessed April 15, 2014, available at www.holisticprimarycare.net/topics/topics-a-g/acupuncture-a-oriental-med/12-the-five-faces-of-adhd-a-chinese-medicine-approach.

49 **supplements, breathing, and other mind-body techniques** Ibid.

50 **IBS is not "all in your head"** "Irritable Bowel Syndrome," National Digestive Diseases Information Clearinghouse website, NIH Publication 13-693, September 2013, updated October 7, 2013, accessed April 15, 2014, available at http://digestive.niddk.nih.gov/ddISeases/pubs/ibs/.

50 **While IBS symptoms can be considerable** Ibid.

50 **Crohn's disease or ulcerative colitis do** Ibid.

50 **gastroenterologists are identifying** Ibid.

50 **substance called 5-hydroxytryptophan** Manocha and Khan, "Serotonin and GI Disorders."

50 **people with IBS** Case-Lo, "IBS and Serotonin."

51 **can't put two thoughts together** "What Is Non-Celiac Gluten Sensitivity?" National Foundation for Celiac Awareness website, accessed April 15, 2014, available at www.celiaccentral.org/non-celiac-gluten-sensitivity/introduction-and-definitions/.

51 **six times the number with CD** Ibid.

51 **in this case, the intestinal lining** Jane Anderson, "Gluten Sensitivity vs. Celiac Disease," About.com, updated March 29, 2014, accessed April 15, 2014, available at http://celiacdisease.about.com/od/glutenintolerance/a/Gluten-Sensitivity-Vs-Celiac-Disease.htm.

51 **If their symptoms improve** Ibid.

51 **attention, irritability, and depression** Ibid.

51 **red flag for undiagnosed CD** Jessica R. Jackson et al., "Neurologic and Psychiatric Manifestations of Celiac Disease and Gluten Sensitivity," *Psychiatric Quarterly* 83, no. 1 (March 2012): 91–102, doi:10.1007/s11126-011-9186-y, accessed April 15, 2014, available at www.ncbi.nlm.nih.gov/pmc/articles/PMC3641836/.

52 **almost 9 percent in boys to 14 percent in girls** Luigi Mazzone et al., "Compliant Gluten-Free Children with Celiac Disease: An Evaluation of Psychological Distress," *BMC Pediatrics* 11, no. 46 (2011), published online May 27, 2011, doi:10.1186/1471-2431-11-46, accessed April 15, 2014, available at www.ncbi.nlm.nih.gov/pmc/articles/PMC3149570/.

CHAPTER 4. DIET-FREE WEIGHT LOSS

54 **promote a state of calm alertness** Elizabeth Somer, *Eat Your Way to Happiness: 10 Diet Secrets to Improve Your Mood, Curb Your Cravings, Keep the Pounds Off* (New York: Harlequin, 2009), 44–45.

54 **increase serotonin production** Ibid.

54 **soothing, appetite-stomping serotonin** Ibid..

54 **stress depletes serotonin in the brain** Daniel G. Amen, "Kava Kava and St. John's Wort,"

accessed April 15, 2014, available at www.grossmont.edu/lifecoach/docs/KavaKavaand
StJohnsWort.pdf.

54   **with reward mechanisms in the brain**   "Brain Basics."

54   **Presto—weight gain**   Julia Reinholz et al., "Compensatory Weight Gain Due to Dopa-
minergic Hypofunction: New Evidence and Own Incidental Observations," *Nutrition and
Metabolism* 5, no. 35 (2008), doi:10.1186/1743-7075-5-35, accessed April 15, 2014, available
at www.nutritionandmetabolism.com/content/5/1/35.

54   **fewer dopamine receptors than the brains**   Gene-Jack Wang et al., "Brain Dopamine and
Obesity," *The Lancet* 357, no. 9253 (February 3, 2001): 354–57, doi:10.1016/S0140-6736
(00)03643-6, accessed April 15, 2014, available at www.thelancet.com/journals/lancet
/article/PIIS0140-6736(00)03643-6/fulltext.

55   **crawling with 100 trillion microbes**   Lal Rup, "The Human Microbiome Project," *Indian
Journal of Microbiology* 52, no. 3 (September 2012): 315, doi:10.1007/s12088-012-0304-9, accessed April 15, 2014, available at www.ncbi.nlm.nih.gov/pmc/articles/PMC3460114/.

55   **influences our moods and even our personalities**   Moheb Costandi, "Microbes on Your
Mind," *Scientific American Mind* (July/August 2012), 23, 32–37, doi:10.1038/
scientificamericanmind0712-32, accessed April 15, 2014, available at www.nature.com
/scientificamericanmind/journal/v23/n3/full/scientificamericanmind0712-32.html.

56   **in ways that are concerning**   "Your Microbes and You: The Good, Bad, and Ugly," *NIH
News in Health,* November 2012, accessed April 15, 2014, available at http://newsinhealth
.nih.gov/issue/Nov2012/Feature1.

56   **led to significant weight gain**   Paul Kudlow, "Ten Parts Bacteria, One Part Human,"
Canadian Medical Association Journal 185, no. 5 (March 19, 2013): 377–78, doi:10.1503/
cmaj.109-4405, accessed April 15, 2014, available at www.ncbi.nlm.nih.gov/pmc/articles
/PMC3602252/; Fritz Francois et al., "The Effect of *H. pylori* Eradication on Meal-
Associated Changes in Plasma Ghrelin and Leptin," *BMC Gastroenterology* 11, no. 37
(2011), doi:10.1186/1471-230X-11-37, accessed April 15, 2014, available at www.biomed
central.com/1471-230X/11/37.

56   **more than those in the human genome**   "Your Microbes and You: The Good, Bad, and
Ugly."

57   **bad bacteria like *Clostridium difficile***   Kirsty Brown et al., "Diet-Induced Dysbiosis of
the Intestinal Microbiota and the Effects on Immunity and Disease," *Nutrients* 4, no. 8
(August 2012): 1095–1119, doi:10.3390/nu4081095, accessed April 15, 2014, available at
www.ncbi.nlm.nih.gov/pmc/articles/PMC3448089/.

57   **life-threatening inflammation of the colon**   "C. Difficile Infection," Mayo Clinic website,
updated July 16, 2013, accessed April 15, 2014, available at www.mayoclinic.org/diseases
-conditions/c-difficile/basics/definition/CON-20029664?p=1.

58   **easier to make themselves at home in your gut**   J. A. Hawrelak and S. P. Myers, "The
Causes of Intestinal Dysbiosis: A Review," *Alternative Medicine Review* 9, no. 2 (June 2004):
180–97, accessed April 15, 2014, available at www.ncbi.nlm.nih.gov/pubmed/15253677.

58   **the diversity and composition of the gut flora**   Les Dethlefsen and David A. Relman,
"Incomplete Recovery and Individualized Responses of the Human Distal Gut Microbiota
to Repeated Antibiotic Perturbation," *Proceedings of the National Academy of Sciences* 108
(Supp. 1, March 15, 2011): 4554–61, doi:10.1073/pnas.1000087107, accessed April 15, 2014,
available at www.ncbi.nlm.nih.gov/pmc/articles/PMC3063582/; "Effects of Antibiotics on
Gut Flora Analyzed," *Science Daily,* published January 9, 2013, accessed April 15, 2014,
available at www.sciencedaily.com/releases/2013/01/130109081145.htm.

58   **bacteria that would otherwise keep us lean**   "Your Microbes and You," *NIH News in
Health,* November 2012, accessed April 15, 2014, available at http://newsinhealth.nih.gov
/issue/Nov2012/Feature1.

58   **about a dozen courses of antibiotics**   Kudlow, "Ten Parts Bacteria, One Part Human."

58   **NSAIDs (aspirin, ibuprofen, naproxen)**   "NSAIDs and Peptic Ulcers," National Digestive Diseases Information Clearinghouse (NDDIC), NIH Publication 10-4644, April 2010,

updated November 27, 2013, accessed April 15, 2014, available at http://digestive.niddk
.nih.gov/ddiseases/pubs/nsaids/#4.

58   **such as lead, cadmium, arsenic, chromium, and mercury**   Marc Monachese et al., "Bio-
remediation and Tolerance of Humans to Heavy Metals through Microbial Processes: a
Potential Role for Probiotics?" *Applied and Environmental Microbiology* 78, no. 18 (September 2012): 6397–6404, accessed April 15, 2014, available at http://aem.asm.org/content/78
/18/6397.full.

58   **bacterial composition of the gut**   Jérôme Breton et al., "Ecotoxicology Inside the Gut:
Impact of Heavy Metals on the Mouse Microbiome," *BMC Pharmacology and Toxicology*
14, no. 62 (2013), doi:10.1186/2050-6511-14-62, accessed April 15, 2014, available at www
.ncbi.nlm.nih.gov/pmc/articles/PMC3874687/?report=classic.

59   **Mice fed the *Lactobacillus rhamnosus* bacterium**   Rebecca Boyle, "Bacteria in Gut Influence Brains of Mice, Soothed by Probiotic Broth," *Popular Science,* posted August 30, 2011,
accessed April 15, 2014, available at www.popsci.com/science/article/2011-08/probiotic
-broth-reduces-stress-mice-researchers-report.

59   **which helps regulate emotional behavior**   Javier A. Bravo et al., "Ingestion of *Lactobacillus* Strain Regulates Emotional Behavior and Central GABA Receptor Expression in a
Mouse via the Vagus Nerve," *Proceedings of the National Academy of Sciences,* 108, no. 38
(September 20, 2011), accessed April 15, 2014, available at www.pnas.org/content/108/38
/16050.full.

59   **not more prone to developing asthma**   H. Bisgaard et al., "Reduced Diversity of the Intestinal Microbiota During Infancy Is Associated with Increased Risk of Allergic Disease
at School Age," *Journal of Allergy and Clinical Immunology* 128, no. 3 (September 2011):
646–52.e1–5. doi:10.1016/j.jaci.2011.04.060, accessed April 15, 2014, available at www.ncbi
.nlm.nih.gov/pubmed/21782228.

59   **a "new, safe, well tolerated and natural treatment"**   Ludovico Abenavoli et al., "Probiotics in Nonalcoholic Fatty Liver Disease: Which and When," *Annals of Hepatology* 12, no. 3
(May-June 2013): 357–63, accessed April 15, 2014, available at www.annalsofhepatology
.com/numeros/2013/ah133_may-june_v12_n3_2013/PDFs/02_133_v12n3_2013
_ProbioticsAlcoholic.pdf.

59   **from their mother's gut via breast milk**   "'Breast Is Best': Good Bacteria Arrive from
Mum's Gut via Breast Milk," *Environmental Microbiology,* news release, published Au-
gust 22, 2013, accessed April 15, 2014, available at www.sfam.org.uk/download.cfm?docid
=F75D8C6C-129B-4A7B-94FCDB081E3F789A.

60   **diseases associated with it, including type 2 diabetes**   Le Chatelier et al., "Richness of
Human Gut Microbiome."

60   **characteristic of virtually all chronic diseases**   Ibid.

60   **a protective role against weight gain**   "Rich or Poor in Gut Bacteria: We Are Not All
Equal Facing Obesity Related Diseases," news release, French National Institute for Agricultural Research, accessed April 15, 2014, available at http://presse.inra.fr/en/Resources
/Press-releases/Rich-or-poor-in-gut-bacteria-we-are-not-all-equal-facing-obesity
-associated-diseases.

60   **Diet can help turn poverty to richness**   Aurelie Cotillard et al., "Dietary Intervention
Impact on Gut Microbial Gene Richness," *Nature* 500, no. 7464 (August 29, 2013): 541–46,
doi:10.1038/nature12506, accessed April 15, 2014, available at www.nature.com/nature
/journal/v500/n7464/full/nature12480.html.

60   **studied the changes in their gut bacteria**   Ibid.

60   **clinical symptoms associated with obesity**   Ibid.

61   **lower the risk of chronic disease**   "Rich or Poor in Gut Bacteria."

61   **the entire group had low genetic diversity**   Le Chatelier et al., "Richness of Human Gut
Microbiome."

61   **and diet can play a significant role**   Ibid.

61   **shift the balance of bacteria in the gut**   Linda Geddes, "Diet Switch Sparks Gut Bug

Revolution in Just 24 Hours," *New Scientist Health,* no. 2947, December 11, 2013, accessed May 12, 2014, available at www.newscientist.com/article/mg22029473.400-diet-switch -sparks-gut-bug-revolution-in-just-24-hours.html#.U07h3zbn-M9.

61   **diverse types and amounts of fiber**   Joanne Slavin, "Fiber and Prebiotics: Mechanisms and Health Benefits," *Nutrients* 5, no 4 (April 2013): 1417–35, doi:10.3390/nu5041417, accessed April 15, 2014, available at www.ncbi.nlm.nih.gov/pmc/articles/PMC3705355/.

62   **betray bacterial "poverty" in your gut**   "Cedars-Sinai Study: Obesity May Be Linked to Microorganisms Living in the Gut," Cedars-Sinai news release, published March 26, 2013, accessed April 15, 2014, available at www.cedars-sinai.edu/About-Us/News/News -Releases-2013/Cedars-Sinai-study-Obesity-may-be-linked-to-microorganisms-living-in -the-gut.aspx.

62   **fibers selectively stimulate the growth**   Ibid.

63   **contains 14 to 25 times more omega-6s**   "Omega-6 Fatty Acids," University of Maryland Medical Center website, reviewed June 17, 2011, accessed April 15, 2014, available at http:// umm.edu/health/medical/altmed/supplement/omega6-fatty-acids#ixzz2xI28oyOb.

63   **high amounts of processed foods**   "Essential Fatty Acids," Physician's Committee for Responsible Medicine website, accessed April 15, 2014, available at www.pcrm.org/health /health-topics/essential-fatty-acids.

63   **Rebalancing this ratio can help support**   "Omega-3 Fatty Acids," George Mateljan Foundation website, accessed April 15, 2014, available at www.whfoods.com/genpage.php ?tname=nutrient&dbid=84.

63   **immune response and cool inflammation**   Bernhard Hennig et al., "Nutrition Can Modulate the Toxicity of Environmental Pollutants: Implications in Risk Assessment and Human Health," *Environmental Health Perspectives,* doi:10.1289/ehp.1104712, accessed April 15, 2014, available at http://ehp.niehs.nih.gov/1104712/.

64   **cookies and crackers, and stick margarine**   "Trans Fats," American Heart Association website, accessed March 15, 2014, available at www.heart.org/HEARTORG /GettingHealthy/FatsAndOils/Fats101/Trans-Fats_UCM_301120_Article.jsp.

64   **linked with bacterial diversity in the gut**   Inés Martínez et al., "Gut Microbiome Composition Is Linked to Whole Grain–Induced Immunological Improvements," *ISME Journal* 7, no. 2 (February 2013): 269–80, doi:10.1038/ismej.2012.104, accessed April 15, 2014, available at www.ncbi.nlm.nih.gov/pmc/articles/PMC3554403/.

64   **an increase in the gluten content**   "Celiac Disease: On the Rise," *Discovery's Edge,* July 2010, Mayo Clinic website, accessed April 15, 2014, available at www.mayo.edu/research /discoverys-edge/celiac-disease-rise.

64   **food manufacturers use wheat gluten**   Donald D. Kasarda, "Can an Increase in Celiac Disease Be Attributed to an Increase in the Gluten Content of Wheat as a Consequence of Wheat Breeding?" *Journal of Agricultural and Food Chemistry* 61, no. 6 (February 13, 2013): 1155–59, doi 10.1021/jf305122s, accessed April 15, 2014, available at www.ncbi.nlm.nih .gov/pmc/articles/PMC3573730/.

65   **22 teaspoons of added sugars**   Rachel K. Johnson et al., "Dietary Sugars Intake and Cardiovascular Health: A Scientific Statement from the American Heart Association," *Circulation* 120 (2009): 1011–20, doi:10.1161/CIRCULATIONAHA.109.192627, accessed April 15, 2014, available at http://circ.ahajournals.org/content/120/11/1011.full.

66   **American Heart Association has set strict limits**   Ibid.

66   **Protein is found in many different foods**   "High-Protein Foods," Stanford Cancer Center website, accessed April 15, 2014, available at http://cancer.stanford.edu/information /nutritionAndCancer/during/highProteinFood.html.

67   **severe bacterial infection *Clostridium difficile***   "C. Difficile Infection," Mayo Clinic website, updated July 16, 2013, accessed April 15, 2014, available at www.mayoclinic.org /diseases-conditions/c-difficile/basics/definition/CON-20029664?p=1.

67   ***C. difficile* infection can cause bouts**   Ibid.

67   **recolonize the sick person's bowel**   "Ohio State's Wexner Medical Center Performing

Fecal Transplants to Treat Serious Intestinal Infections," The Ohio State University Comprehensive Cancer Center website, news release, published July 1, 2013, accessed April 15, 2014, available at http://cancer.osu.edu/mediaroom/releases/Pages/Ohio-State's-Wexner-Medical-Center-Performing-Fecal-Transplants-To-Treat-Serious-Intestinal-Infections.aspx#sthash.SFGeXrGm.FQpqSoWu.dpuf.

67   **found FMT significantly more effective**   Els van Nood et al., "Duodenal Infusion of Donor Feces for Recurrent *Clostridium difficile,*" *New England Journal of Medicine* 368 (January 31, 2013): 407–15, doi:10.1056/NEJMoa1205037, accessed April 15, 2014, available at www.nejm.org/doi/full/10.1056/NEJMoa1205037#t=article.

69   **gut bacteria may adapt to that glut**   A. N. Payne et al., "Gut Microbial Adaptation to Dietary Consumption of Fructose, Artificial Sweeteners and Sugar Alcohols: Implications for Host-Microbe Interactions Contributing to Obesity," *Obesity Reviews* 13, no. 9 (September 2012): 799–809, doi:10.1111/j.1467-789X.2012.01009.x., accessed April 15, 2014, available at www.ncbi.nlm.nih.gov/pubmed/22686435.

CHAPTER 10. SEVEN STRESS SOOTHERS FOR A HAPPY GUT

143   **our times of biggest stress coincide**   "Fact Sheet on Stress," National Institute of Mental Health website, accessed April 16, 2014, available at www.nimh.nih.gov/health/publications/stress/index.shtml.

143   **stress is the body's automatic physiologic reaction**   "Stress: Fight or Flight," Massachusetts General Hospital, Benson-Henry Institute for Mind-Body Medicine website, accessed April 16, 2014, available at www.bensonhenryinstitute.org/index.php/stress-fight-or-flight.

143   **cells in the nervous and endocrine systems**   "How Cells Communicate During Fight or Flight," University of Utah Health Sciences, Genetic Science Learning Center website, accessed April 16, 2014, available at http://learn.genetics.utah.edu/content/cells/fight_flight.

144   **the automatic part of the stress response**   "Understanding the Stress Response," Harvard Health Publications website, accessed April 16, 2014, available at www.health.harvard.edu/newsletters/Harvard_Mental_Health_Letter/2011/March/understanding-the-stress-response.

144   **"switched on" for weeks, months, or even years**   "Good Stress, Bad Stress: Research identifies health impact of different responses," *Stanford Medicine Newsletter,* Fall 2012, accessed April 16, 2014, available at http://stanfordmedicine.org/communitynews/2012fall/stress.html.

144   **involves every system in the body**   "Defining Stress," UCLA Center for East-West Medicine website, accessed April 16, 2014, available at http://exploreim.ucla.edu/mind-body/defining-stress/.

144   **slow them down, leading to constipation**   Lisa Tams, "Stress and Health—Part 2," Michigan State University Extension website, published October 8, 2013, accessed April 16, 2014, available at http://msue.anr.msu.edu/news/stress_and_health_part_2.

145   **THREAT AHEAD. STOP DIGESTING**   "Why Being Mindful Matters," University of Minnesota website, accessed April 16, 2014, available at www.takingcharge.csh.umn.edu/explore-healing-practices/food-medicine/why-being-mindful-matters.

145   **discomfort ranging from heartburn to gas**   Tams, "Stress and Health—Part 2."

145   **inflammatory bowel disorders in people predisposed**   "Learning How Stress May Affect the Digestive System Will Be Topic of Free UCLA Lecture," news release, University of California at Los Angeles, June 3, 2002, accessed April 16, 2014, available at http://newsroom.ucla.edu/portal/ucla/Learning-How-Stress-May-Affect-3244.aspx.

145   **study published in *The American Journal of Gastroenterology***   Charles N. Bernstein et al., "A Prospective Population-Based Study of Triggers of Symptomatic Flares in IBD,"

American Journal of Gastroenterology 105 (September 2010): 1994–2002, doi:10.1038/ajg .2010.140, accessed April 16, 2014, available at www.nature.com/ajg/journal/v105/n9/full /ajg2010140a.html.

145 **stress may predispose a person** "Stress," University of Maryland Medical Center website, reviewed January 30, 2014, accessed April 16, 2014, available at http://umm.edu/health /medical/reports/articles/stress.

145 **increased their vulnerability** Carpenter, "That Gut Feeling"; Michael T. Bailey et al., "Exposure to a Social Stressor Alters the Structure of the Intestinal Microbiota: Implications for Stressor-Induced Immunomodulation," *Brain, Behavior, and Immunity* 25, no. 3 (March 2011): 397–407, accessed April 16, 2014, available at www.ncbi.nlm.nih.gov/pmc /articles/PMC3039072/.

147 **Consciously slowing your breathing** "Relaxation Techniques for Health: An Introduction," National Center for Complementary and Alternative Medicine, NCCAM Publication D461, August 2011, updated February 2013, accessed April 16, 2014, available at http://nccam.nih.gov/health/stress/relaxation.htm.

147 **to benefit their physical and spiritual well-being,** Vishvender Singh et al., "Applied Aspect of Pranayama in Maintaining Health," *Ancient Science of Life* 32 (Supp. 1, December 2012): S94, accessed April 16, 2014, available at www.ncbi.nlm.nih.gov/pmc/articles /PMC3800977/.

149 **seventy-five women with IBS** S. A. Gaylord et al., "Mindfulness Training Reduces the Severity of Irritable Bowel Syndrome in Women: Results of a Randomized Controlled Trial," *American Journal of Gastroenterology* 106, no. 9 (September 2011): 1678–88, doi:10.1038/ajg.2011.184, accessed April 16, 2014, available at www.ncbi.nlm.nih.gov /pubmed/21691341.

150 **People all over the world have inhaled** "Aromatherapy," University of Maryland Medical Center website, updated May 7, 2013, accessed April 16, 2014, available at https://umm .edu/health/medical/altmed/treatment/aromatherapy.

151 **a 2013 study published in The Journal of Neuroscience** "A Shot of Anxiety and the World Stinks," *University of Wisconsin-Madison News,* September 24, 2013, accessed April 17, 2014, available at www.news.wisc.edu/22154.

152 **divided thirty people with reflux** R. Dickman et al., "Clinical Trial: Acupuncture vs. Doubling the Proton Pump Inhibitor Dose in Refractory Heartburn," *Alimentary Pharmacology and Therapeutics* 26, no. 10 (November 2007): 1333–44, accessed April 16, 2014, available at http://onlinelibrary.wiley.com/doi/10.1111/j.1365-2036.2007.03520.x/full.

153 **regular prayer, along with general stress management** Christopher G. Ellison et al., "Religious Involvement, Stress, and Mental Health: Findings from the 1995 Detroit Area Study," *Social Forces* 80, no. 1 (September 2001): 215–49, accessed April 16, 2014, available at www.jstor.org/discover/10.2307/2675537?uid=3739592&uid=2&uid=4&uid=3739256& sid=21103874374937.

154 **yoga classes a week for three months** "Yoga for Health," National Center for Complementary and Alternative Medicine, NCCAM Publication D472, May 2008, updated June 2013, accessed April 14, 2014, available at http://nccam.nih.gov/health/yoga/introduction .htm.

155 **Hatha yoga combines physical poses** "Yoga," National Center for Complementary and Alternative Medicine, modified March 21, 2014, accessed April 14, 2014, available at http:// nccam.nih.gov/health/yoga.

155 **massage slows heart rate** "Massage Therapy: What You Knead to Know," *NIH News in Health,* July 2012, accessed April 15, 2014, available at http://newsinhealth.nih.gov/issue /jul2012/feature2.

CHAPTER 11. THE 21-DAY BELLY FIX WORKOUT

159   **Regular exercise does a body good**   "Physical Activity Improves Quality of Life," American Heart Association website, reviewed March 22, 2013, accessed April 16, 2014, available at www.heart.org/HEARTORG/GettingHealthy/PhysicalActivity/StartWalking/Physical-activity-improves-quality-of-life_UCM_307977_Article.jsp.

159   **Reduces risk of heart disease**   "Exercise and Physical Fitness," MedLinePlus, accessed April 16, 2014, available at www.nlm.nih.gov/medlineplus/exerciseandphysicalfitness.html#cat22.

159   **well-documented ability to reduce stress**   "Physical Activity Improves Quality of Life."

159   **make the neurotransmitter norepinephrine**   "Exercise and Depression," *Harvard Health Publications,* accessed April 16, 2014, available at www.health.harvard.edu/newsweek/Exercise-and-Depression-report-excerpt.htm.

160   **promotes proper bowel movements**   "Constipation," MedLinePlus, updated September 2, 2012, accessed April 16, 2014, available at www.nlm.nih.gov/medlineplus/ency/article/003125.htm.

160   **the National Cancer Institute estimates**   "Physical Activity and Cancer Risk," Cancer.net, reviewed September 2013, accessed April 16, 2014, available at www.cancer.net/navigating-cancer-care/prevention-and-healthy-living/physical-activity/physical-activity-and-cancer-risk.

160   **Men and women who run have**   Paul T. Williams, "Incident Diverticular Disease Is Inversely Related to Vigorous Physical Activity," *Medicine and Science in Sports and Exercise* 41, no. 5 (May 2009): 1042–47, doi:10.1249/MSS.0b013e318192d02d, accessed April 16, 2014, available at www.ncbi.nlm.nih.gov/pmc/articles/PMC2831405/.

160   **20–30 minutes of moderate exercise**   "Exercise Improves Symptoms in Irritable Bowel Syndrome," news release, University of Gothenberg, the Sahlgrenska Academy, updated January 21, 2011, accessed April 16, 2014, available at www.sahlgrenska.gu.se/english/news_and_events/news/News_Detail/exercise-improve-symptoms-in-irritable-bowel-syndrome.cid974984.

160   **regular exercise can help keep your gut**   "Physical Inactivity Worsens GI Symptoms in Obese People," news release, *EurekAlert!,* published 10/3/2005, accessed April 16, 2014, available at www.eurekalert.org/pub_releases/2005-10/aga-piw092905.php.

160   **moderate exercise may lower**   Hamed Khalili et al., "Physical Activity and Risk of Inflammatory Bowel Disease: Prospective Study from the Nurses' Health Study Cohorts," *British Medical Journal* (2013); 347, doi:http://dx.doi.org/10.1136/bmj.f6633, published November 14, 2013, accessed April 16, 2014, available at www.bmj.com/content/347/bmj.f6633?view=long&pmid=24231178.

161   **All of its benefits accrue from activity**   "Physical Activity and Arthritis Overview," Centers for Disease Control and Prevention website, updated November 23, 2013, accessed April 16, 2014, available at www.cdc.gov/arthritis/pa_overview.htm.

161   **can lead to heartburn and GERD**   E. P. de Oliveira and R. C. Burini, "The Impact of Physical Exercise on the Gastrointestinal Tract," *Current Opinion in Clinical Nutrition and Metabolic Care* 12, no. 5 (September 2009): 533–38, doi:10.1097/MCO.0b013e32832e6776, accessed April 16, 2014, available at www.ncbi.nlm.nih.gov/pubmed/19535976.

161   **gastrointestinal bleeding are common side effects**   H. Peters et al., "Potential Benefits and Hazards of Physical Activity and Exercise on the Gastrointestinal Tract," *Gut* 48 (2001): 435–39, doi:10.1136/gut.48.3.435, accessed April 16, 2014, available at http://gut.bmj.com/content/48/3/435.full.

161   **Extreme exercise can also weaken**   Ibid.

163   **Kegels can improve urine leakage**   "Pelvic Floor Muscle Training Exercises," MedLinePlus, updated June 18, 2012, accessed April 16, 2014, available at www.nlm.nih.gov/medlineplus/ency/article/003975.htm.

163   **tighten and move up**   Ibid.

164   **fatigue the muscles and increase urine leakage**   Ibid.

164   **incorporate Kegels into your normal routine**   "Pelvic Muscle Exercises," National Association for Incontinence website, accessed April 16, 2014, available at www.nafc .org/stress-incontinence/index.php?page=pelvic-muscle-exercises&gclid=CMv32o_gzrw CFWUOOgod0WAAag.

165   **can improve your health _and_ your quality**   "Physical Activity and Heath: The Benefits of Physical Activity," Centers for Disease Control and Prevention website, updated February 16, 2011, accessed April 16, 2014, available at www.cdc.gov/physicalactivity/everyone /health/.

165   **Blood flow to the muscles and lungs increases**   "Fitness," Mayo Clinic website, updated March 4, 2014, accessed April 16, 2014, available at www.mayoclinic.org/aerobic-exercise /ART-20045541?p=1.

165   **improve your health in a multitude of ways**   "Why Strength Training?" Centers for Disease Control and Prevention website, reviewed February 24, 2011, accessed April 16, 2014, available at www.cdc.gov/physicalactivity/growingstronger/why/.

166   **estimated that a pound of muscle takes up**   "Physical Activity: Frequently Asked Questions," Centers for Disease Control and Prevention website, reviewed February 24, 2011, accessed April 16, 2014, available at www.cdc.gov/physicalactivity/growingstronger/faq/.

166   **maintain a healthy weight**   "Why Strength Training?"

166   **can linger in body fat for decades**   "Polychlorinated Biphenyls (PCBs) and Your Health," Wisconsin Department of Health Services website, revised March 17, 2014, accessed April 16, 2014, available at www.dhs.wisconsin.gov/eh/fish/PCBlink.htm.

166   **your core muscles include more than just the abs**   Christie Matheson, "Strengthening and Protecting Your Core Muscles," NYU Langone Medical Center website, reviewed November 2013, accessed April 16, 2014, available at www.med.nyu.edu/content?ChunkIID =13836.

168   **lower back, hips, and abdomen to work together**   "Core Exercises," Mayo Clinic website, reviewed October 1, 2011, accessed April 16, 2014, available at www.mayoclinic.org/core -exercises/ART-20044751?p=1.

169   **endurance from 40 percent to 100 percent**   "U.Va. Researcher Studies and Promotes Realistic Exercise Plan," news release, _Inside UVA Online,_ February 2–8, 2001, accessed April 16, 2014, available at www.virginia.edu/insideuva/2001/04/gaesser.html.

Index

ABOUT THE AUTHOR

TASNEEM "DR. TAZ" BHATIA, M.D., is a board-certified physician, the founder and medical director of the Atlanta Center for Holistic and Integrative Medicine, and a fellow at the Arizona Center for Integrative Medicine of the University of Arizona (led by Dr. Andrew Weil). Best known as Dr. Taz, M.D., she has been featured on *The Dr. Oz Show, Today, Live with Kelly and Michael,* CNN, and the Weather Channel and was a contributing editor and columnist for *Prevention.* She currently serves as a health expert for Mom Corps YOU and Cancer Treatment Centers of America and is an associate professor at Emory University. She resides in Atlanta, Georgia.

ABOUT THE TYPE

This book was set in Granjon, a modern recutting of a typeface produced under the direction of George W. Jones, who based Granjon's design upon the letter forms of Claude Garamond (1480–1561). The name was given to the typeface as a tribute to the typographic designer Robert Granjon.